The Alexander Technique
in Everyday Life

(The need for illustration) forces the philosopher or teacher to give to the world practical procedures which may be applied to the actual activities of life, instead of theoretical conclusions which too often have no practical bearing on life. This formula, I venture to predict, will prove to be more and more the rule and not the exception as we progress towards a plane of constructive, conscious guidance and control.

F.M. Alexander

JONATHAN DRAKE

The Alexander Technique in Everyday Life

Thorsons
An Imprint of HarperCollins*Publishers*

Thorsons
An Imprint of HarperCollins*Publishers*
77–85 Fulham Palace Road,
Hammersmith, London W6 8JB
1160 Battery Street,
San Francisco, California 94111–1213

First Published by Thorsons 1991 as *Body Know-How*
This revised edition published 1996
10   9   8   7   6   5   4   3   2   1

A catalogue record for this book
is available from the British Library

ISBN 0 7225 3290 3

Printed in Great Britain by Scotprint Ltd., Musselburgh, Scotland.

Contents

Acknowledgements

I am extremely grateful to Marjory Barlow, Misha Magidov, John Naylor, Shelley Stokes and Mervyn Waldman for their scrutiny of the manuscript. Their comments and advice greatly sharpened my thinking and have helped to clarify the presentation of material in this book; none the less, I take full responsibility for the content. I am also indebted to Sue Lloyd for her assistance in improving the readability of the text and to Jane Asher for her comments on the section on swimming.

I was very fortunate indeed to have the contrasting tendencies of body use so expertly and patiently demonstrated by Dorothea Magonet; and thanks are due also to Peter Reynolds Studios, Northampton, for their technical expertise.

Without the initial teaching and inspiration of Patrick Macdonald and Misha Magidov I might have stopped asking questions long ago. My pupils have also prodded me gently with their challenging questions.

Rahula Books and Patrick Macdonald kindly granted permission to use quotations from *The Alexander Technique: As I See It*.

Finally – and not least! – many thanks to my family, and particularly Angela, for bearing with me during much re-working of the manuscript, and for her constant encouragement and guidance.

Foreword

My introduction to the Alexander Technique was Tinbergen's 1973 oration as Nobel Prize winner for Medicine/ Physiology, and in 1977 I began lessons in the Technique. Having worked in experimental physiology for 35 years I am increasingly impressed by the importance of Alexander's discoveries.

Our muscles constitute a fascinating organ, comprising over a third of our body mass. Most people would regard muscle as simply being there for keeping us upright, enabling us to move and providing strength to do things. Muscles are much more; they are part of an important sense organ (the 'sixth sense' as described by the nineteenth century physiologist Sir Charles Bell – the proprioceptive or kinaesthetic sense). Muscles provide our means of communication of information and emotion: externally, via speech (generated by muscle), facial expression and body posture; and internally by the contribution muscles make to our emotional state (the lax muscles of depression and the tense muscles of anxiety or anger).

F.M. Alexander called attention to his discovery that we, in the modern world, have cut ourselves off from our sixth sense, and hence have cut ourselves off from the optimum use of our muscles for posture, movement, communication and emotional states or moods.

How do we regain the sixth sense and re-establish optimum muscle use? It is only by being prepared to spend time on and pay attention to our muscle state, and, by allowing new patterns of muscle control to be established, to enable anti-gravity muscles to function simply and without unnecessary added contractions (or co-contractions). The skilled hands of a teacher not only help to awaken the muscle sense in a pupil but also help to stimulate more appropriate muscle patterns. The learning of these sensory and motor experiences is essentially non-verbal. Nevertheless, it is a great help to thinking people to have some idea of what is going on and what to expect.

In this respect Jonathan Drake's book makes a very useful contribution. In clear and simple prose he explains the basic principles of the Alexander Technique. He describes a range of procedures one can do and observe oneself doing in association with the essential inputs from the skilled hands of a teacher. Not only is the book marked by its practicality (applying the

Alexander Technique to working at a computer keyboard or driving a car) but also by plentiful illustrations of good 'technique' in action. These two features make the book invaluable to anyone interested in the Alexander Technique or anyone undertaking lessons in it.

David Garlick B.Sc., MB, BS, Ph.D.
Senior Lecturer
School of Physiology and Pharmacology
University of New South Wales

Introduction

The Alexander Technique in Everyday Life is for anyone who wants to know how to improve their body-use. Through applying the insights of the Alexander Technique, it is possible to avoid a good deal of the undue stress, strain, pain and fatigue of daily life.

When people first hear about the Alexander Technique, they usually ask what it is they have to 'do': aren't there any physical exercises? The answer is: most emphatically not. Physical exercise routines – even the very latest 'fitnetics' program! – often embarked on to compensate for the static postures associated with modern sedentary living, contribute to the very problems they are supposed to solve. What Alexander showed is actually needed is a radical re-thinking of how we perform all those *everyday* activities that we take so much for granted.

The grace and beauty of well-coordinated movement and posture are a delight to observe and experience. These things come naturally to animals – who rely mainly on instinct – and to decreasing numbers of people in the developed world. We acquire the basic skills of coordination spontaneously when we are very young, but as we grow through childhood, most of us begin to deteriorate. Surveys of 18-year-old students at colleges of physical education and speech and drama – who should be better than average – showed that 80 per cent had substantial or severe postural defects on beginning their course.[1] The condition of the students who followed the remedial exercises prescribed worsened during their course. Only those who had received Alexander lessons significantly improved.

It is a sad commentary on modern living that this bodily misuse has become so much the norm that most of us are hardly aware of it. Unwittingly we abuse our bodies, which have a great capacity for adaptation – especially when we are young. Sooner or later, however, we pay the price with a whole host of stress-related disorders, and we suffer the disappointments of not being able to achieve goals in life which are important to us. Body-misuse is a primary cause.

F.M. Alexander's discovery

F. Matthias Alexander (1869–1955) – the founder of the Alexander Technique – discovered the key to restoring our natural co-ordination and thereby improve how we function in all aspects of our lives.

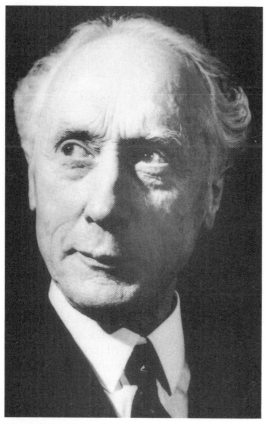

Fig. 1 F.M. Alexander

He concluded that the majority of us need to consciously re-learn how to use our bodies in a more efficient way during the activities of daily living. The fundamental principles he described which govern good body-use are still largely unknown, ignored or misunderstood by many 'experts' in the field – whether doctors, physiotherapists, sports coaches, fitness trainers or performing arts teachers (the reason for which will become clear during the course of this book).

The aim of this book

The Alexander Technique in Everyday Life aims to bridge the gap between the basic ideas of the Alexander Technique and their practical application. The Technique is occasionally presented in a way which fosters mystique or which can make Alexander's insights seem quite inaccessible. However, a reviewer of Alexander's first book, *Man's Supreme Inheritance*, described his methods as 'systematised common sense'; it is this frequently elusive common sense – applied to daily life – which this book aims to detail.

The first part of the book tells of Alexander's extraordinary story and the increasing relevance of his observations, concepts and experiments to our own experience. The second part is concerned with application. Certain procedures are described and illustrated in detail – a teacher will ensure you understand them correctly. These can help you improve the way you carry out all the various activities of daily living: from simple tasks, such as vacuuming, to the most complex of skills, such as playing a musical instrument.

Alexander and his teachers have always been hampered by the limitations of language; moreover, intellectual knowledge is no substitute for the subtle (and sometimes confusing) experience of the new coordination which can be given to you by a properly-trained teacher. You wouldn't expect to go very far in learning a musical instrument without skilled help; and your body is your most important instrument!

Sometimes, however, it may not be possible to consult a teacher and it is hoped that the thoughtful reader, by understanding certain facts, will be helped to avoid some of the worst aspects of body-misuse.

Pupils having Alexander lessons with me often would remark: 'I see the point of what you're showing me in the lesson, but when I'm on my own I find it difficult to remember how to put it into practice in my daily life. Can you recommend a suitable book for me?' I had to concede that while there are a number of excellent books on the concepts of the Alexander Technique, there was not one that would provide them with the detailed, practical guidance they sought.[2]

When I first began learning the Technique, I was fortunate to have teachers who had the manual skills to give me powerful, direct and accurate sensory experience of good body-use. Nevertheless, I now believe that my own progress in learning the Alexander Technique would have been more satisfactory had I understood the relevance of certain things more clearly at an earlier stage. The assumption seemed to be made that if the pupil learns to 'get out of the way' so that correct experiences of improved coordination can be imparted repeatedly, he or she will eventually find out how to apply the Technique to their daily life.

That did not happen very readily for me. What I would have liked early on was a framework in which to understand better how to apply the Technique to my life.

My story

In common with many people starting lessons in the Technique, I didn't at first appreciate the extent to which I was in a mess. I played squash to a reasonable standard and I thought my coordination couldn't be so bad. I didn't comprehend then that you might be very competent in one sphere and yet be in great trouble generally. I couldn't understand why my teacher advised me – at least for a while – to give up my sporting exertions and my yoga exercises! Gradually, though, my perception sharpened. I came to see how I was distorting myself through these activities, and a glimmer of understanding began to dawn. As Alexander teachers will frequently say: 'I have been finding out ever since.'

Before I came to the Technique I had had a rigid middle back and scolioses (sideways twists in the spine). Chronic chest infections

and pneumonia in childhood, the carrying of heavy newspapers slung across my back on a paper round as a teenager and the one-sided development encouraged by racket sports – these, amongst other causes, played their part. Years of school and university studying added to the excessive tension and pulling down in my body.

In medical school, my studies in anatomy were devoted to the corpse. In later years, having graduated and left medicine, as a student of the Alexander Technique, I learnt to give the most detailed attention to the dynamics of the body in movement, and its poise – or lack of it.

I owe an incalculable debt to the Technique and its teachers for many of the insights I have gained into improving my health and well-being over the past decade. I believe that the Technique has helped me avoid disabling back problems and has probably reduced the risks of serious internal disorders. I seem to be able to thrive on higher levels of stress than I was able to as a struggling medical student. Above all, it has given me considerably more confidence in coping with new situations, and greater learning skills.

Who can benefit from this book?

There is much advice for anyone wanting to cope better with their daily life; Alexander's insights can speak to all of us – whatever our background and whatever we do. *Designed primarily to be used as a Workbook for people already taking Alexander lessons*, it will also be a useful source of information for:

- someone thinking of taking Alexander lessons;
- anyone wanting to: take more responsibility for their own health and well-being; avoid undue fatigue, strain and pain from

everyday living; develop poise and confidence and thrive on reasonable levels of stress; improve their body form, image and coordination;

- teachers, musicians, actors, dancers, athletes and sportsmen/women;
- anyone wanting to enhance their learning and mastery of skills;
- anyone suffering from back and neck pain; frozen shoulder, tennis elbow, 'regional pain syndrome' or 'repetitive strain' injuries in musicians and keyboard operators; various forms of arthritis – especially osteoarthritis of the spine, hip and knee; stress-related or psychosomatic disorders – headaches, breathing difficulties, gastro-intestinal problems and hypertension;
- those wishing to aid rehabilitation after pregnancy, illness, injury or accident;
- anyone coping with depression and anxiety;
- anyone wanting some guidance in the design and use of the work and leisure environment, such as the use of appropriate chairs, desks, etc.

PART ONE

The basic ideas

An individual is in the best health only when the body is so used that there is no strain on any of its parts. This means that when standing the body is held fully erect, with no strain on the joints, bones, ligaments, muscles or any other structures. There should be adequate room for all the viscera, so that their function can be performed normally.

Goldthwaite *et al.*, *Body Mechanics*

CHAPTER 1

What is good body-use?

That mind and body work together so that they cannot easily be separated is now more generally accepted, but it was a remarkably bold proposition for F.M. Alexander to make in his time. He employed the expression 'use of the self' to denote the quality or style of coordination of the mind/body in *all* activities of daily life.

While a well-coordinated person can be readily distinguished from a badly-coordinated one, subtle differences may not be so obvious. The untrained eye may be deceived. For instance, the apparent lightness of classical ballet dancers in often achieved by great physical effort. Gymnasts gain much of their exceptional suppleness at the expense of forced bending of joints. Both groups suffer greatly from injuries; and degenerative joint changes frequently develop in early and middle-adult life.

A few fortunate individuals manage to retain supremely good body-use naturally for longer than most of us. Dancers like Astaire and Baryshnikov, pianists Rubinstein and Horowitz, boxer Muhammed Ali and tennis player Steffi Graf come to mind.

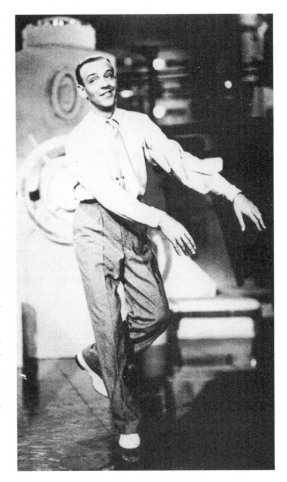

Fig. 2 Fred Astaire – the immortal! Such lightness and ease of movement. (Photo: Rex Features)

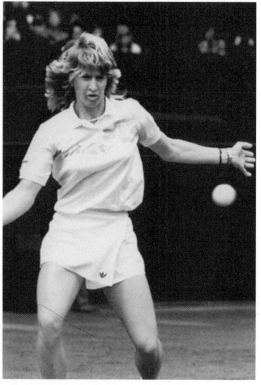

Fig. 3 *Steffi Graf, Wimbledon, 1987. A superb athlete, showing the powerful co-ordinated use of her legs and whole body to produce her classic crunching forehand drive.* (Photo: Rex Features)

The features of ideal movement

Do you know how to analyse the quality of a voluntary movement? Here is a useful way:

- *Absence of effort*: only what needs to be done, is done. There is economy of movement, no internal resistance, absence of effort and no disturbance of breathing. The movement could be repeated many times without strain and fatigue setting in.
- *Reversibility*: it should be possible to slow, stop and reverse the movement (apart from jumping!). There should be no jerkiness, tremor or instability. When a move-

ment can be performed very slowly – and with ease – great delicacy, control, speed and power are then possible.[1]

To illustrate this, observe how much undue effort most of us make when walking. If you stand in front of a large mirror and take a few steps *very slowly*, you can begin to see what happens when you walk. See how uncontrolled you are, and how heavily your weight falls onto your front heel as you step forwards. You may be surprised to realize how wobbly your balance is (especially if you try to walk backwards!). If you observe how other people walk, you will see any number of individual variations. In common though, is a lack of balance and fluidity of movement. We don't think about *how* we walk; after all, most of us learnt to walk at about one year old! In Part 2 you will see how it is possible, through the Alexander Technique, to learn how to improve walking – or any activity – even if it is set in a long-established pattern.

Over-specialization of body-use

Since the industrial revolution, the range of movements most of us perform in the course of our lives has narrowed. We tend to be relatively immobile – seated – often making repetitive movements. Housework involves much bending down and predisposes us to the development of a hump in the back. In our leisure time it is all too easy to slump, exhausted, in front of the TV. The other extreme is to dig the garden all weekend or take up some form of vigorous exercise.

Unfortunately most forms of exercise tend to consolidate the very habits we are trying to change. This can be extremely harmful. An estate agent who used to play squash to compensate for occupational stress periodically had a seized-up back. He went for treatment to get him back on the road, but no one warned him that his posture and coordination were appalling. Finally a lumbar disc prolapsed, part of it was removed and he came to see me in terrible pain, his lower back in spasm. Osteopathy in his case hadn't helped. He

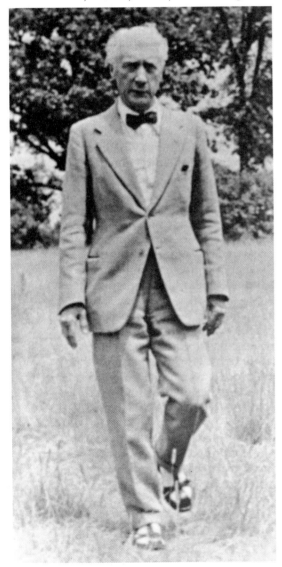

Fig. 4 Alexander walking. Note the light, expansive movement and free use of all the joints in his legs.

wasn't able to make the necessary changes in his life style to give himself the chance of avoiding further surgery and he was heading for a total disc removal and a spinal fusion. I warned him that this would probably not stop his pain altogether and would almost certainly lead to compensatory problems elsewhere in his spine. His only hope in the long term was to deal with the main cause of his difficulties – his misuse of himself.

Doctors use labels such as 'repetitive strain injury', 'tenosynovitis', and 'regional pain syndrome' for the increasingly common problems suffered by computer operators and musicians. (Frozen shoulder, tennis elbow and writer's cramp are manifestations of the same kind of phenomenon.) The usual medical explanation for this range of conditions is *over*-use and the treatments prescribed include rest, pain-killing drugs, operations or a change of occupation.

The origins of the Alexander Technique

A century ago, the young Australian actor, F.M. Alexander, had a vocal problem; his medical label was also over-use. He had been increasingly troubled by hoarseness on stage. Finally his voice failed him utterly in the middle of a recital. His doctors gave him the usual advice – rest or have operative treatment (there being only mild inflammation of his vocal cords). Rest restored his voice – for a while – but under the stress of performance it would worsen again.

Alexander, however, passionately wanted to pursue an acting career. He reasoned that it must be something he was doing to himself that was causing his difficulty (with which his medical advisors had to agree), and since no one could tell him exactly what he was doing, he resolved to find out for himself. In the course of his self-enquiry it became clear to him that his trouble was due less to over-use of his vocal mechanism, more due to *mis*-use of himself as a whole.

Eventually he discovered how to prevent the misuse and he had no further difficulty with his voice. He had suffered from chronic illnesses since childhood; and in recovering his voice, his general health improved. When he taught other actors what he had learnt about the use of the voice, they frequently reported a general improvement in their functioning.

He came to the conclusion, therefore, that he had stumbled on something of far greater significance than a solution to the particular problems of vocalization. *He had found the key to a method by which coordination can be fundamentally improved – which can benefit all aspects of our functioning.*

How we have gone awry

Alexander came to see the problem in evolutionary and anthropological terms. He

Fig. 5 Slack stomach muscles are usually produced by slumped posture.

Fig. 6 Tightening of stomach muscles and buttocks leads to general stiffening.

Fig. 7 Good use and balanced muscle tone corrects unduly bulging abdomen.

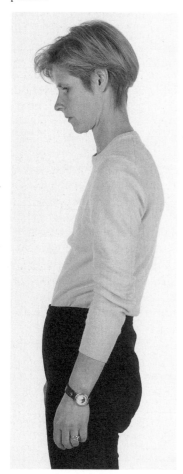
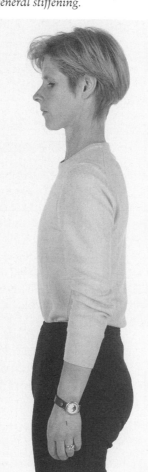
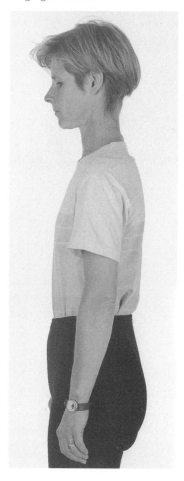

taught that we can no longer rely entirely on subconscious control of our coordination in the rapidly-changing world we have created. We require more *conscious* control of ourselves than that needed by the hunter-gatherers or even the early farmers.

It is obvious that there is no single cause for the almost universal misuse which is now evident in most peoples, but all of the following factors play a part:

- *Static positions and repetitive activities* (including exercise routines); these put extra strain on a body that is going out of balance.
- *Emotional stresses* can lead to distortions in body structure, which in turn can limit the range of emotions someone can experience. For instance, a depressed person often pulls down into themselves, producing a lack of vitality which can feed their emotional problems – depression becomes a habit.

  Our sense of personal identity is bound up with the particular ways we hold ourselves. Body language conveys, often subconsciously, messages about how we want others to respond to us.
- *Imitation*; we copy the significant people in our lives as we grow up – parents, teachers, popular musicians, fashion models and so forth. We can often catch ourselves 'mirroring' the posture of someone we are with, especially if we wish to appear in any way sympathetic to them. Beset by so many images of poor coordi-

nation in the media and in our daily lives, the aesthetic of ideal body form *in movement* – now seen largely in terms of muscular development or the fashionable amount of fatness or thinness – is all too easily lost.

- *Physiological compensation*, e.g. in pregnancy, accidents, injuries, and illnesses; through an injury to one part of the body or through prolonged bed-rest in chronic illness, the whole system can go out of balance. Compensations may become habitual and operate when no longer necessary. As we grow older we tend to go more 'out of kilter'.

Whatever the reasons may have been for the development of our individual patterns of misuse, the Alexander Technique can be used to help get us out of difficulty. In addition, more and more people are using Alexander's insights to help prevent serious trouble in the future, and to achieve their life goals in the most efficient and effective ways. Age is no bar to learning the Technique. Older pupils may take longer but are sometimes better motivated than younger ones, for whom it can be all too easy to ignore the possible consequences of present actions!

Before we find out how to set about improving our body-use, more needs to be explained about the key to coordination which Alexander called the 'primary control'.

CHAPTER 2

The primary control

Alexander did not make an extensive study of anatomy or physiology, but his books demonstrate that over the years he had marshalled a useful working knowledge of biological principles to give support to his observations and arguments. An important factor in Alexander's ability to re-discover the key to coordination – as he saw it – must have been the keen powers of observation he developed in childhood, through a love of horses and the wild game of the Australian bush. *Perhaps this enabled him to see the essentials which a detailed knowledge of human biology might have caused him to miss.* As Tinbergen, who devoted half of his Physiology and Medicine Nobel Prize Oration in 1973 to an account of the Technique, said:

This story of perceptiveness, of intelligence, and of persistence, by a man without medical training, is one of the true epics of medical research and practice.[1]

John Dewey, American philosopher and educationalist, who wrote the forewords to three of Alexander's books – and whose thinking had been greatly influenced by his lessons with Alexander – stated:

After studying over a period of years Mr Alexander's method in actual operation, I would stake myself upon the fact that he has applied to our ideas and beliefs about ourselves and our acts exactly the same method of experimentation . . . that has been the source of all progress in the physical sciences.

Alexander's early observations and experiments

Since no one could tell Alexander exactly how he was interfering with his voice – apart from a tendency to make audible gasping sounds between phrases – he set up a system of mirrors to compare the way he recited with his normal speaking. What he noticed was an exaggerated tendency to stiffen his neck and retract his head, as well as to raise his chest and to hollow his lower back. This involved a marked contraction and shortening of his stature, and harmful pressures on his vocal cords and all his internal organs. Later he realized that this pattern of undue tension spread throughout his body right down to the tips of his toes – he would grip the stage floor with his feet. He came to see that this pattern of misuse was present all the time, in varying degrees, depending on how much stress he was experiencing.

At first he tried to change everything at once – without success. The key to his whole coordination, he discovered after some time, was the orientation of his head on his neck. If he could control that, then the misuse of the rest of his body was reduced.

The sort of misuse he observed in himself is so prevalent that we are not usually aware of it in ourselves or others. However, if you observe the movement of getting into and out of a chair – which involves a big change of position – you can see the misuse demonstrated in a striking way. Place yourself at an angle to a mirror and slowly get up and down. You will probably see your head

Fig. 8 A common form of misuse begins with the neck stiffening, the head retracting, the chest raising and the lower back hollowing.

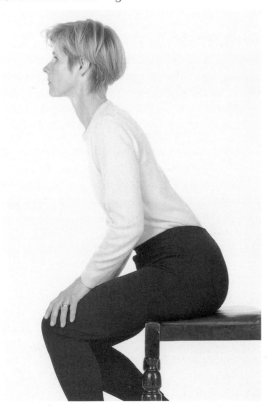

pulling back and down into your shoulders as you sit down or stand up (occasionally you will see just the opposite – the chin pulling down towards the chest). The significance of this movement – repeated many times in the course of the day – is that it demonstrates the way in which most of us tend to misuse ourselves in *all* our everyday actions.

The startle response

Supporting evidence for Alexander's claim that the neck/head balance is of crucial importance to our whole coordination is the 'startle response'. This shows how the reaction to a certain kind of stress distorts the body. In the psychology laboratory, a subject is monitored for the distribution of muscular tension produced in response to a loud, unexpected sound. The spread of excessive tension begins in the neck and the head retracts into the shoulders. You can see daily examples of this on the TV screen as political and religious demagogues adopt similar kinds of postures as they strive to move their audiences. And as people age, they tend to shrink into their shoulders – the cumulative effect of a lifetime of unrelieved stress responses.

The primary control

Alexander used the phrase 'the primary control' to describe the particular relationship between neck, head and back/torso (which will be abbreviated hereafter to NHB relationship) which influences the coordination of the rest of the body. If the head is freely and delicately balanced on top of the neck, so that the torso can expand instead of being shortened and narrowed, the coordination of the limbs and the whole body is facilitated.

Let's consider this balancing of the head on the neck. The head weights 3–4 kilos in

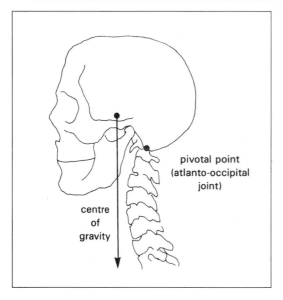

Fig. 9 Centre of gravity of the head is carried forward of its pivot on the neck.

an adult – equivalent to three bags of flour – quite a heavy weight supported on a narrow column. In babies the weight of the head is proportionately even greater in relation to the rest of the body; yet the mechanism for control of the head develops quite easily in normal circumstances. The centre of gravity of the head is actually slightly forwards and upwards of its point of balance on the first neck (cervical) vertebra.(You may have noticed how the head of someone in an upright position nods forward when they fall asleep.) If you ask someone to nod their head gently and you then enquire where he or she thinks the movement takes place, the presumption is usually that the head–neck joint is lower down and further back than it actually is. In fact it is almost at the level of the ears. The consequence of this kind of misconception is that the neck is stressed most of the time. The potential for independent movement of the head on the neck and its implications for coordination as a whole will not then be realized.

The balance of the head on the neck is maintained by the coordinated action of all the neck muscles, but principally by the tone in muscles at the *back* of the neck. Now there are two groups of muscles which help to stabilize head balance. In most people the larger group is far too active and tends to pull the head back and *down* through attachments to the shoulder blades and collar bones. These big muscles can be seen standing out when excessive effort is being made or when the startle response is invoked.

If you come to a standing position from sitting or its reverse, and you wrap your hand around the back of your head – with your little finger at the base of the skull and your thumb resting on the top of your shoulder blade – you can feel this happening. As you get up or sit down you will almost certainly notice your hand span reduced as your neck arches – bending mostly at its base – and you will feel those big muscles contracting. This is an unnecessary waste of effort and sets up harmful contractions throughout the body.

There is a smaller group of muscles – the sub-occipital muscles – which lie deeper and are attached to the base of the skull and the first and second cervical vertebrae and which, if their function is not usurped by the larger muscles, maintain the delicate balance of the head on the neck.

Since Alexander drew attention to the importance of the primary control, physiological knowledge has increased enormously and provides corroboratory evidence for Alexander's claims.[2] It is now known that these sub-occipital muscles contain the highest density of special sensory organs (proprioceptors) of any muscle in the human body – even compared with the muscles of the hand. These proprioceptors are responsible for recording changes in muscle tension; and in the joints, they contribute to the sense of where one part of the body is in relation to other body parts.

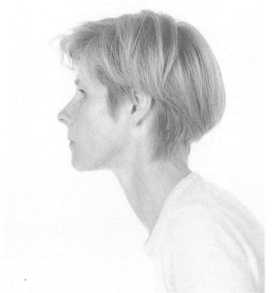
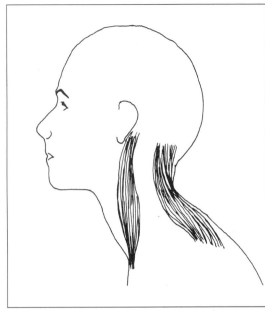

Fig. 10 Overworking larger neck muscles.

Fig. 11 Larger neck muscles passing from base of skull down the neck onto torso.

Figs. 12 and 13 Smaller sub-occipital muscles responsible for maintaining delicate head balance.

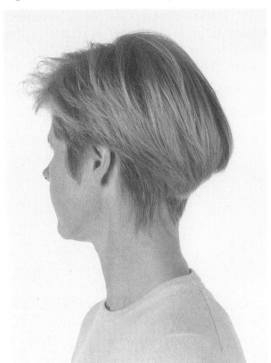
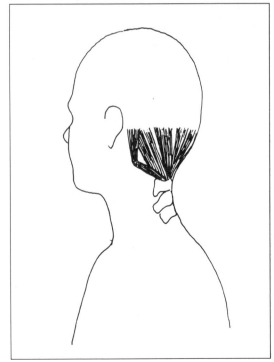

They are part of our *kinaesthetic* sense (our vital and neglected sixth sense). If there is excessive activity in the larger muscles, discrimination between different kinds of movement of the head becomes difficult or impossible.

When the primary control functions as it should, coordination takes on a totally different quality. Movement becomes smoother, easier and lighter, and excessive muscular contractions and pressures on joints are reduced. To a trained pair of hands feeling the tone of a well-coordinated body, the spine takes on an extraordinary quality like a flowing liquid – completely different to the heaviness felt when a person pulls down into themselves.

Body structure can be thought of in terms of a stacking system, one part loaded on top of the next part and so forth. However, when the body is well-coordinated, the relation of body parts to each other can be more accurately described as a suspension system; it is as though the person is a puppet, the head suspended from a string and the rest of the body supported by the head. All the joint surfaces then tend to separate away from each other.

To improve coordination as a whole and in all its aspects, it is thus necessary to restore the proper relationship between neck, head and back – the primary control. The method that Alexander devised to do this will be described next.

CHAPTER 3

How to change

You cannot change and yet remain the same, though this is what most people want.

Patrick J. Macdonald

Change involves carrying out an activity against the habit of life.

F.M. Alexander

Force of habit and faulty kinaesthesia

At first Alexander thought it would be a comparatively easy matter to restore the proper NHB relationship, even though he could see by now that the vast majority of people showed a derangement of the primary control. The difficulty he found he was up against in making fundamental change turned out to be due to two major and related factors.

To avoid the pulling back of his head, Alexander did what most of us would try to do – the opposite. He tried to *put* his head forward and up. He found, though, that he either stiffened his neck and fixed his head in position or he put it forward and down. In short, he succeeded only in modifying the original misuse – the changed pattern was merely 'a different kind of badly'. Force of

habit, he came to recognize, was considerably more powerful than he had bargained for. The stress of recitation, even in the privacy of his own room, always seemed to invoke the pattern of misuse that he had come to associate with his vocal trouble, however much he tried to avoid it.

At times he believed he had succeeded in avoiding the pulling back of his head. However, when he checked for confirmation in his mirrors, there was the incontrovertible evidence that he was not actually doing what he felt he was doing. Thus the other important barrier to real change – and closely linked to habit – was his reliance on his kinaesthetic (feeling) sense to organize his body, this being largely a subconscious process, and very often faulty.

Faulty kinaesthesia has two aspects. Sometimes there has been so much misuse in a part of the body that the brain stops registering what is occurring; chronically-hunched shoulders are one example. Secondly, the brain may misinterpret the information received; many examples of this will be given in Part 2. *The brain appears to confuse the habitual pattern of use with the correct, ideal pattern. This serves to underline the difficulty of making change without the aid of a teacher.* Alexander's classic illustration of this kind of delusion is his account of a young crippled girl brought by her mother to him for an opinion. When he straightened out her twisted body, the girl turned to her mother and exclaimed 'in an indescribable tone, "Oh! Mummie, he's pulled me out of shape."'[1]

And so, after many unsuccessful attempts trying to get it right, the first breakthrough came when Alexander realized that *the new pattern he needed to bring about would feel wrong and uncomfortable to him at first, precisely because it was not his usual way of doing things.* For a simple demonstration of this, try the following. Put this book down for a moment and cross your arms in your usual way; then, uncross them and cross them the other way. How does the other way feel? If you are not ambidextrous, you will probably find that the alternative manner of folding your arms feels awkward, uncomfortable, wrong. (And you might even have had to look down to see exactly how to cross your arms!) There is no necessary reason why a slightly different way of doing something should feel so wrong, yet to most of us it does.

Further investigation showed Alexander that by the time he had begun to recite, the malcoordination was well established. An example of this is the experience of driving a car on a long journey, or being in a desperate hurry to get somewhere while stuck in a traffic queue! A niggling pain frequently starts up in the base of the neck and across the top of the shoulders. However much you try to roll the head about, the only way to relieve the tension is to get out of the car and rest or change your activity.

The next and crucial breakthrough came when he put the question: at what point does the faulty pattern of misuse begin to get a hold? The answer to his question came – in front of the mirrors – when he noticed that *once he had committed himself to the idea of reciting,* he could see his body *getting set* for the activity of reciting. He realized, therefore, that he must change his thinking. At the point at which he intended to do something – which re-stimulated the old pattern – he must say 'no' to the habitual response. He called this process *inhibition,* the necessary first step in undoing old habit patterns.

Inhibition: what it is and what it is not

Confronted with a familiar stimulus, we are often driven to respond automatically. A cat stalking its prey and delaying its attack until the most opportune moment is an example of inhibition in the animal kingdom – partly learnt, but mostly instinctual. The hotheaded youth who goes ahead with an action he is later going to have cause to regret, contrasts with the calm reflection of a more mature person deciding that it is better not to act in a given situation! Assertiveness training involves, amongst other things, learning that you have as much right to say 'no' as 'yes', when you are put on the spot.

It is easy to forget that in any situation, however limited the actual range of possibilities, we always have some element of choice. Of course, the habitual response (R_h) may be the appropriate one to a familiar stimulus (S). Sometimes it is not. It might be better – if only we allowed ourselves to stop and reflect – not to respond at all (R_0). Or there may be any other number of responses which merit consideration $(R_{1,2,3}$ etc). Logically, then, at each moment we have these possible choices:

$$S \rightarrow R_h$$
$$S \rightarrow R_0$$
$$S \rightarrow R_{1,2,3} \text{ etc}$$

So, the first step in facilitating change is to delay or prevent the habitual response. This is not easy. Alexander insisted that *'the conscious mind must be quickened'*. It is interesting to note, in this connection, the possible relevance of recent work by the physiologist Libet.[2] He showed that the brain takes about 3/10ths of a second to get ready for a voluntary action, but that it is only in the next 2/10ths of a second – during which time volition reaches a conscious level – that the otherwise automatic progression to the activation of muscle can be countermanded.

Inhibition thus provides an opportunity to choose your response from the range of possibilities right up to the last moment you have to commit yourself to action. This withholding of action, or *non-doing*, gives us the chance of regaining our poise by becoming more aware of the subtle ways in which we may be interfering with the efficiency of performing a movement. Alexander maintained that if you can learn to inhibit your habitual responses, remarkable changes can be made relatively quickly and easily; otherwise, conflict is produced by trying to overlay a new response on top of the old one.

More often than not, our main concern is to achieve our ends even if such *end-gaining* – as Alexander called it – leads to exaggerated effort and tension. Inhibition prevents us from running ahead of ourselves; instead, if we decide to commit ourselves to the process – the *means-whereby* as Alexander called it – we can achieve our ends more economically.

It will be clear by now that Alexander did not use 'inhibition' in the same sense that it is employed in psychotherapy. In Alexander's sense, someone who habitually blocks their feelings is just as much in need of inhibition as someone who flies off the handle at the earliest opportunity. It should be possible to delay the habitual response; perhaps for a moment, perhaps indefinitely. There is then room for creative spontaneity because old, reactive responses can be avoided.

Giving directions

Once Alexander was able to inhibit his habitual response to the idea of reciting, he was still left with residual patterns of misuse. All the time, of course, messages are passing from the brain to the body to control its responses; and even to voluntary muscles this is mostly a subconscious process. To undo further these patterns of misuse – and to maintain his general co-ordination while reciting – he devised certain *directions* (or orders, as Alexander frequently called them) to be given to the primary control. (See table at the bottom of the page.)

These directions are *conscious* messages from the brain to the parts of the body concerned to prevent faulty use and to promote coordination (the subordinate directions to the limbs will be described in detail later). In time – *with the help of a competent teacher's hands* – these directions will not just be given verbally but will gain in content and clarity of experience.[3]

Effects of subconscious habits:	Preventive directions to be given:
stiffened neck	let the neck be free
head retracted into shoulders	to let the head go forward and up
back shortened and narrowed	to let the back lengthen and widen

More explanation of these directions will be given in Part 2. For the moment, notice particularly the word 'let'; it means that the directions are not to be carried out directly, muscularly. To be sure, a kind of activity occurs, but it is so small as to take place almost below the sense register. And the directions are to be given in the proper sequence, as written on page 27. In time they operate together, all at once. It is analogous to learning to drive a car: initially the proper flow of actions is ill-timed, often out of sequence, and the car may stall, but as skill develops its operation becomes smooth and automatic.

Illustrations of directed movement

How is it that thoughts can lead to significant changes in physical activity? The eminent neuro-physiologist Sir Charles Sherrington pointed out how all nervous pathways from the brain end in muscle. To help you understand what giving directions involves, the example given by Macdonald (Alexander's distinguished senior teacher) may be helpful.[4] Hold out a forefinger and then wiggle it about. Now take hold of your forefinger with the fingers of your other hand and gently pull. When you release your fingers, there should be the experience of the forefinger stretching itself which continues for a while as you again move the forefinger; directed movement – compared with ordinary movement – has this subtle but all-important quality of ease, expansiveness and freedom.

The difference between a directed action and the ordinary tensed action, when *some* effort is required, can be strikingly demonstrated as follows. With the help of a partner, hold your arm out in front of you a little below shoulder level, palm upwards, and ask your partner to place one hand on your upper arm just above your elbow, their other hand underneath your forearm by your wrist. Their task is to bend your arm at the elbow. At first your intention should be to resist their attempt to bend your arm at the elbow as they (*steadily*, so no one injures themselves!) increase the pressure. It helps if you grit your teeth, clench your fist and generally tighten everywhere!

Next approach this task in a quite different way. Release the tension in your jaw and throat, uncurl your fingers and be quite clear that all you need to think is to let your arm lengthen out of your shoulder out to the tips of your fingers. Continue to allow this lengthening process in your arm despite your partner's attempt to bend it.

You will find that your partner will probably be quite unable to make any change in the directed arm, whereas the stiffened arm will be relatively easy to flex. If you swop round, you will be able to feel the marked difference in power in your partner's arm under the alternative conditions. (Note that the directed arm is not 'relaxed': it does not hang limply at the side. Alexander was very much opposed to relaxation as most people understand it – a form of collapse – which prevents well-coordinated movement.)

The physiological reason for this extraordinary difference in response is that muscle at a certain length is able to exert more power than over-shortened muscle. How is this example relevant to the NHB (neck-head-back) relationship? The same principle applies, but it takes longer for directions to the primary control to produce such a dramatic effect; over a hundred joints are involved in the NHB relationship. For large changes to occur, little ones must take place first and, in time, learning to direct the primary control properly will allow the necessary changes to take place.

Concentration versus attention

Alexander thought that concentration *per se* was harmful when it excludes the ability to be alert to other things going on at the same time. The notion of consciously directing certain aspects of ourselves in activity seems very strange at first, especially as we are used to relying on subconscious control of our coordination. This seems all the more so if you can recall the experience you may have had of trying to perform an action *while* thinking about it. Your coordination will have worsened and you may have lost your balance! In this situation, though, you are usually trying to interfere *directly* with movement. The processes of inhibition and direction-sending – properly understood – have nothing to do with that kind of control; on the contrary, thought is used in an indirect way to facilitate the 'undoing' which is necessary to allow actions to do themselves.

When first learning the Technique, most people pass through a phase of awkward self-consciousness. This 'thinking in activity' need not displace sense data coming from the outside world – nor the awareness of other thoughts and feelings. Rather, the aim is to strike a better balance between the need to focus your attention selectively as well as to be able to scan the wider field of consciousness. For example, I can be aware of and direct my walking *and* talk to a companion *and* avoid stumbling on a brick on the kerbside, *while* noticing that a bus is bearing down on us *and* that we had better wait before crossing the road!

Summary

We need to recognize the full extent to which we are creatures of habit. We should also understand that any direct attempt to change our habits by using the same mechanism that has become untrustworthy – namely kinaesthesia – inevitably produces a 'different kind of badly' (which makes it harder to eradicate than the original problem).

Instead, Alexander's solution is to learn how to become aware of and inhibit our faulty patterns of use. They can be replaced gradually with new patterns through the process of giving directions – allowing the primary control to operate more as it should. At first this will only be possible with relatively simple activities, but eventually it can be extended to the most complex activities.

The more we learn to apply the Technique, the more accurate our kinaesthesia becomes. What our restored kinaesthetic sense can alert us to is when and how we are going wrong. We then have the opportunity to improve the way we carry out our daily activities.

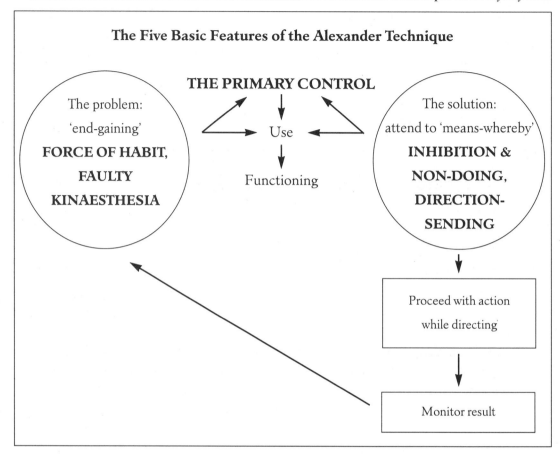

The Five Basic Features of the Alexander Technique

THE PRIMARY CONTROL

The problem: 'end-gaining' **FORCE OF HABIT, FAULTY KINAESTHESIA**

Use

Functioning

The solution: attend to 'means-whereby' **INHIBITION & NON-DOING, DIRECTION-SENDING**

Proceed with action while directing

Monitor result

PART TWO

Putting it into practice

Everyone wants to be right, but no one stops to consider if their idea of right is right.

F.M. Alexander

When anything is pointed out, our only idea is to go from wrong to right in spite of the fact that it has taken us years to get wrong: we try to get right in a moment.

F.M. Alexander

Generally speaking it takes people a lot of thinking and hard work, even with the aid of a teacher, to get anything worth having.

P.J. Macdonald

Applying Alexander principles to daily activities

Real change can take place once you understand that you are not going to transform years of misuse overnight. This goes against the whole cultural imperative which Tom Wolfe memorably called 'the burning itch to grab it now!' Instead, your first aim should be to find out exactly what you are doing which may be causing you difficulty or discomfort, or which interferes with your functioning; and you should seek to understand how your 'doing' is created by your intentions.

Any desire you might have to get everything right immediately should be channelled into a willingness to work patiently through the steps necessary for effective change to take place. You will be learning to travel in a certain direction rather than striving for an end-point which really does not exist. Be prepared to experiment – don't be afraid to do the 'wrong' thing sometimes! – and you will be much more likely to make progress.

Part 2 contains detailed instructions for applying Alexander principles to daily activities. *It is important to realize that you will need the assistance of a teacher to ensure you translate correctly the information given.* You will be reminded to inhibit and to give directions constantly; but where the text would become tedious with repetition, I have occasionally omitted to prompt you. Don't forget!

The accompanying photographs were chosen to try to capture 'directed' activity, which is contrasted with the usual tendency to contract in movement. Look at the photographs carefully and try to understand what is required, but do not try to imitate them directly: you are a different size and shape. Moreover it is not a matter of position but quality of coordination, and still pictures can only partly convey this inner dynamic of movement.

People often ask what to expect in learning the Alexander Technique. Some of the most commonly-asked questions – and my attempts to answer them – now follow.

★ ★ ★

It's all very well what you suggest, but how can I find the time to learn the Alexander Technique?

This is the paradox: the more stressed you are, the more you need to deal with the stresses; and yet the less you may think you can do anything about it. The level of stress you can thrive on is very much an individual matter and this can be relatively high for short periods. However, unless you rest and renew yourself there is the long-term risk of sliding down a slippery slope – beginning with fatigue and neurotic symptoms, and ending up with exhaustion and psychosomatic breakdown.

Won't the Technique ever become automatic?

When this question is asked, the penny has usually begun to drop. One of Dr Barlow's pupils reportedly burst out, 'Oh I see, this is a life sentence!' Patrick Macdonald, who had his first lesson from Alexander when he was 10 years old, said, on his 75th birthday: 'The first 65 years are the worst!!'

The point is that you would not expect to play a musical instrument or a sport at all well unless you applied yourself to it for some considerable amount of time. And the efficiency with which you do anything and everything depends on the central instrument: the primary control. Improve that, and you lay the proper foundation for everything that you do. The Alexander Technique has been described as a pre-technique for all activities. Dewey claimed:

It bears the same relationship to education that education itself bears to all other human activities.

Do Alexander teachers think about their own body use all the time?

They aim to in their waking hours and no, they don't entirely succeed – they are only human! Even with three years of almost daily work on a professional training course and their own work on themselves, they are not perfect. As Alexander said: 'Don't you realise that if you get perfection today, you will be further away from it than you have ever been?'

When you make your first attempts to observe yourself in activity you will find that many minutes – sometimes hours – will pass while you are absorbed in whatever you are doing, or simply distracted. It may only be pain that reminds you to pay attention!

The more that you begin to observe your own body use, the more you will notice how frequently and how much you are misusing yourself. This will be very disconcerting at first and most Alexander pupils in their early days – with the odd relapse from time to time – contract what Macdonald calls 'Alexander's gloom'. This is the growing realization of the amount of the work that may need to be undertaken to solve particular difficulties, and to the extent that it is a realistic assessment of the problem, awareness of it is to be welcomed – if only reluctantly!

This process of observation is very similar to the Zen practice of mindfulness of simple, daily tasks and what Gurdjieff meant by 'self-remembering', except – most importantly – it includes an awareness enhanced by more accurate kinaesthetic information.

How much time should I set aside for the Alexander Technique?

In theory, no special time need to be set aside: Alexandrian 'thinking in activity' can be applied from moment to moment as you go about your daily life. In practice, however, everyone can benefit from spending some minutes in the lying-down releasing position daily (see page 38).

When you awake, don't fall out of bed on the buzz of the alarm clock! Give yourself a few minutes to remind yourself that you have a neck, head and back and that they should be encouraged to be in a certain relationship to each other. Then attend to how you shower, wash, brush your teeth and so on. Each day is a new beginning! You will find it easier to be more attentive for the rest of the day if you get off to a good start.

I can't possibly think of everything at first. Where should I begin?

One suggestion is to draw up a list – perhaps over a week – of all the kinds of activities you tend to do. Grade the commonest activities according to degree of difficulty, discomfort or pain experienced. Begin by giving particular attention to one or two of the less demanding daily activities before tackling something more ambitious.

In Part 2, procedures are described which point to what is required in order to improve body use in most activities. You will make more progress in applying the Technique if you take a little time (it need only be two or three minutes) in exploring one or two of these procedures – after being introduced to them by your teacher – perhaps after a lying-down session. To have no aim in mind other than the procedure itself will help you to understand how much work is to be done to improve your coordination in your daily activities.

What does 'thinking in activity' actually require me to do?

It means, first of all, to begin observing how you carry out those everyday activities which are so easily taken for granted. Thinking in activity does not require you to become anxiously watchful in a stilted, stiff kind of way! Before initiating an action, give yourself a pause (it need only be a fraction of a second) so that you have the best chance of recovering your poise and freedom of response. You will then be able to think more clearly about how you are going to carry out the activity.

As well as giving directions prior to an action, they should also be given while performing the action. This is very difficult at first and lessons with a competent teacher will help considerably. Part of the difficulty is to think of several things at once without worsening your coordination. In time, though – rather as in learning to drive a car – you will be able to give the directions in the proper sequence and all at once, during activity. They will then inform the movement. For example, in relation to sexual activity, increased awareness of tension in the body – whether good or faulty – allows your response to a greater degree to be under your control.

Would it be helpful to visualize the directions?

You should be very cautious about using imagery. Alexander did not generally advocate it – nor his senior teachers – because it can become a substitute for the clarity of thinking in activity which needs to be undertaken. To imagine yourself to be light, for example, is likely to make you try to feel it out, rather than creating the conditions which will enable the lightness to come about. Another example is the way that someone will usually try to pull their head up and stiffen the neck if you ask them to imagine a string gently pulling the top of the head upwards. In particular circumstances – in a lesson, for instance – the appropriate use of an image *at a certain point* may help the pupil to allow change, that they may have been blocking, to take place.

Direction-giving is a concrete, precise and subtle activity. In lessons the teacher will give you the experience of the directions operating in movement. On your own, aim to give the directions in the way indicated by the teacher. In time you will experience on your own more accurate sensations of body use.

How can I discover what I am doing?

You will need some form of objective feedback because kinaesthetic sensations are almost certainly not trustworthy and our capacity for self-delusion is almost boundless! The teacher will point out in a mirror –

as appropriate – discrepancies between what you *feel* is happening and what is actually taking place. Alexander used mirrors to work it out for himself and as you learn what to look for, you will also find them of great help. Video is the modern alternative and has obvious advantages over mirrors!

How do I know whether I am improving?

You cannot measure progress in the way you can in learning a language, for instance. The Technique is not about amassing and manipulating information, more about learning to acquire self-control through shedding undue tension. I remember being struck by the title of a book which I came across some years ago – 'Zen Mind, Beginner's Mind'. The more I understand about the Technique, the more amazed I am by how little 'doing' is actually required in most activities. In this respect you always go back to the beginning.

As you progress, you will become more 'present' for longer periods of time. Parts of your body become more 'alive' and you start to understand how they work in relation to each other. For instance, you experience more overall sense of freedom where your head balances on top of your neck. You start to sense the release and separation that should take place at the hip joints between the legs and the torso. Movement becomes freer and lighter. Skills you used to struggle with, you can make steady headway with. You should generally experience less pain and discomfort.

After I had my first few lessons in the Technique, I never again found myself trapped in the grip of that intractable nagging pain at the base of the neck and across the shoulders that plagues many drivers. I had only the minimal understanding of how much I pulled my head back and down into my shoulders, yet that awareness was suffi-cient to begin to dissolve this chronic pattern. I also used to sit for hours at a time in the kind of slumped sitting position that can be seen in most offices and schools. Now if I sit like this it feels immediately unpleasant; and after a few minutes, it becomes quite uncomfortable.

After the initial euphoria of making some change has worn off, you may find yourself slipping back into old patterns if you have a particularly stressful time. Rather than using that experience as an opportunity to beat yourself with a stick, remember that early on you will make compromises, but aim to compromise yourself less as time goes on.

I've been lying down regularly and trying to work on myself but I wonder if I'm doing the 'right' thing? Recently my back has been aching more.

There are three reasons why this may be happening. The first reason is that you may be trying too hard to *do* the directions. Do not force them and remember that the directions to the primary control begin with letting the neck be free. Allow a pause between one set of directions and the next. If this causes a shift in the position of the head on the books when lying down, the chances are that you are forcing the directions. Check that you are not interfering with your breathing or fixing your gaze. Be aware of the sights and sounds around you.

The second reason is that a part of the back which has been chronically tense may be releasing. Information from the affected muscles and soft tissues registers in the brain and you may experience nagging pain. This may pass off quite quickly; sometimes it is more stubborn. You should consult your teacher to determine what is happening.

The third reason is that you may be using muscles once again which have been under-used. Any discomfort in this case should only be temporary.

Why do I feel awkward with this new way of using myself? I don't seem to be able to sit, stand and walk anymore without it feeling wrong!

We often worry unduly about what other people may notice about us. We forget that most people are more often than not preoccupied with themselves!

There is a kind of halfway-house early on. When you first begin lessons you may be in pain yet in one sense you may be quite comfortable with what you do because it is habitual! As you find out more, you begin to realize how much is wrong. You can't easily go back because now you know something you didn't know before. Be patient; in time your new manner of use will feel more comfortable to you and, as you improve, you will be less concerned with temporary feelings of awkwardness or discomfort. Once more, the guidance of a teacher is invaluable.

Have there been any developments in the way Alexander's Technique has been taught since his death?

This is a subject of some controversy in the Alexander world: the 'conservatives' claim that the clarity of his teaching is in danger of being lost; the 'progressives' argue for the need for fresh teaching perspectives.

My viewpoint is that Alexander's essential discoveries stand complete and unchallenged: furthermore, none of his teachers have been able (save, perhaps, the late Patrick Macdonald) to match or surpass his consummate manual skill in conveying 'direction'. One interesting development is from American teachers Barbara and William Conable[1] who, following on from Marjory Barstow's example, have furthered our understanding of the 'lost sixth sense' by identifying common 'mapping errors'. By this they mean the notion that some of our malcoordination stems from assumptions – usually erroneous and unexamined – about the skeleton and how it is articulated. For example, if you have some vague idea that your hip *joints* are located at the level of the hip *bones*, you will bend from the nearest joints – that is, in the lower back. Your subjective map wins out and you won't use your body in accordance with its design: this will create undue stress, strain and degenerative changes in the musculo-skeletal system over time.

CHAPTER 5

On the importance of lying down

Whenever I get the urge to exercise, I lie down until it passes off.

G.K. Chesterton

This quotation was used in a book on exercising: its author took the view that such a remark showed a most deplorable attitude to the virtues of exercise! In an important respect, though, Chesterton is right. If we are badly-coordinated, mechanically-repeated, fast movements – as in most forms of exercise – are likely to emphasize the conditions that are already present and will make us even worse off. What all of us can benefit from is *making a short period of lying down during the day an essential part of every day.*

Why a daily lying-down routine?

At the end of a busy day we are measurably shorter than we were at the beginning – by half an inch, on average, and sometimes by as much as one inch or more. This loss of height is due to our response to gravity – all the more marked as we get older – whether we spend most of our days sitting or engaged in heavy manual work. Muscles become shortened, joints jammed together

and fluid is squeezed out of the intervertebral discs. They tend to flatten, reducing the spaces between the bones (vertebrae) in the back. The biologist D'Arcy Thompson described out potential fate thus:

Man's slow decline in stature is a sign of the unequal contest between our bodily powers and the unchanging force of gravity which draws us down when we would fain raise up. We strive against it all our days, in every movement of our limbs, in every beat of our hearts. Gravity makes a difference to a man's height, and no slight one, between the morning and the evening; it leaves its mark in sagging wrinkles, drooping mouth and hanging breasts; it is the indomitable force which defeats us in the end, which lays us on our death bed and lowers us to the grave.[1]

In fact we can slow down and mitigate some of the ravages of this aspect of the ageing process. Through adequate sleep and regular periods of rest as recommended, fluid is re-absorbed into the discs and they retain their size and shape for longer during the day.

An important property of these discs is to give resilience and elasticity to the supporting function of the backbone. If the spine as a whole retains its proper length and alignment these discs can withstand great pressure. It has been estimated by scientists studying the bio-mechanics of the spine that the vertebrae would be the first structure in the spine to shatter under a colossal downward pressure. The secret of the discs' strength lies in their semi-fluid centre. However, when the spine is distorted and the proper length is lost, the fibrous outer shell of the disc is vulnerable to shearing forces; it may tear and allow the contents to extrude. Nerves running close are then subjected to pressure, producing the sciatic pain experienced by someone with a prolapsed disc.

Furthermore, a period of lying down allows some 'undoing' of the muscular tensions acquired earlier in the day. Biorhythm studies in human beings show approximately 3–4 hour cycles of alertness, followed by short drowsy periods. There is some evidence that these drowsy periods permit fatigued muscle fibres to renew themselves. If we continually struggle to keep going at such times, we will eventually find it very difficult to release chronically-tensed muscles.

Daily lying down is as important for our general health and well-being as brushing our teeth is for avoiding dental problems. It enables us to choose not to respond to the pressures of daily life for a short while – pure inhibition! When there is nothing (or next to nothing) to 'do' and we arrange ourselves in the lying down releasing position to be described shortly, we can become more aware of how much tension we have created: neck and shoulder tensions can be released – the back assumes more of its proper length and shape – and pressure is taken off the joints.

If this lying-down position relieves otherwise constant back pain (and there is no other serious condition present), most sufferers can expect significant relief if they learn to improve their body-use in daily activities.

Fig. 14 Pressure on the discs squashes them; allowing the spine to lengthen restores them.

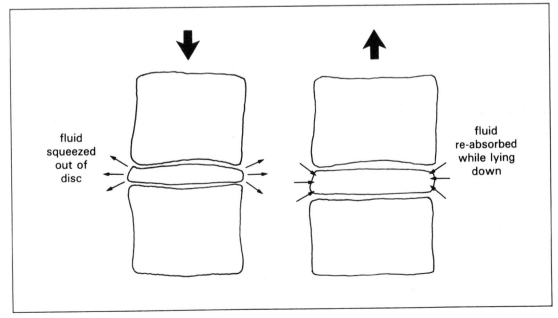

fluid squeezed out of disc

fluid re-absorbed while lying down

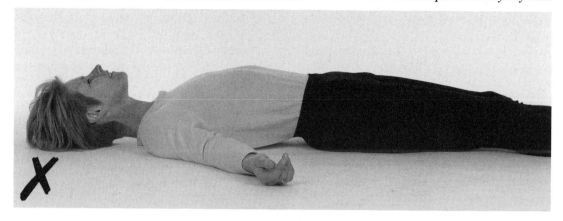

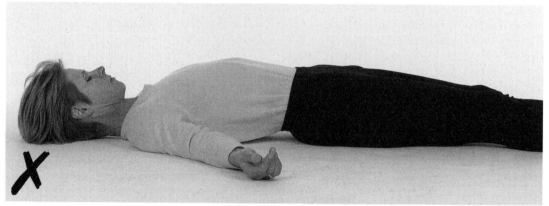

Figs. 15 top and 16 above 'Relaxation' position showing residual tension in neck and back muscles.

Fig. 17 below Lying-down releasing position.

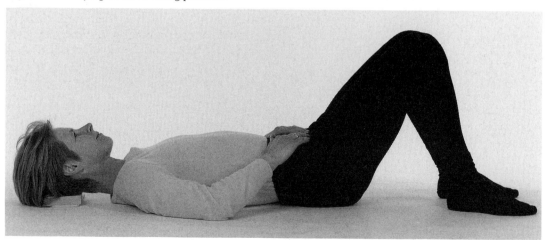

When should I lie down?

Ideally lie down early afternoon. Many cultures take a siesta, but such a prolonged rest is not usually necessary. Allow yourself at least 10–20 minutes (sometimes half an hour or more will be beneficial, if you are especially stressed or fatigued). If you have a desk job, run through the reasons why it might not be possible to find time at work to lie down, and ask yourself whether they are reasonable objections!

Late in the afternoon or early evening a 5–10 minute lie-down may again be welcome. (If it is really not possible to find the space at work, this may be the time when you will have your main lying-down session.) You are also recommended to rest in this way for a few minutes before getting out of bed in the morning to renew your connection with the NHB relationship; and to remind yourself to start the day as you mean to carry on!

Limitations of the most commonly-used relaxation position

Lie down on a firm but comfortable surface – a carpeted floor is most suitable, or a folded blanket on a harder surface – your arms at your sides, legs stretched out. Observe how much of your back is in contact with the floor and be aware of any sensations of undue tension in your body. You will almost certainly notice that your lower back arches off the floor, your head pulls backwards onto the floor and the back of your neck will probably feel a little uncomfortable – unless you have got used to lying in this way! (*Fig. 15*). With the palms upwards and arms close to the sides, the chest is raised and the shoulders pulled back. Note the similarity to the relaxation positions recommended in yoga and certain relaxation techniques. It is often suggested that the chin should be tucked in to stretch out the back of the neck, but this only encourages the harmful habit of contracting the front of the throat (*Fig. 16*).

The lying-down releasing position

Placing some support under the head prevents it from pulling back, and tension in the back of the neck can be released. The lower back can then begin to ease as well. If you bend your knees so that they point up towards the ceiling – about a shoulder's width apart, feet flat on the floor – you will find more of your back closer in contact with the floor (*Fig. 17*).

In this position you should aim to be almost entirely passive physically – letting the floor and books support you – but, with the teacher's help, the aim is to be active mentally, to facilitate the release and separation of parts of the body away from each other.

Height of head support
A small pile of paperback books can be used to provide a firm but comfortable support for the head. You will need enough support to stop the head pulling back yet not so much that the chin is pushed towards the chest and the throat constricted: the aim is to find a neutral and released balance of the head on the neck.

If you are having Alexander lessons your teacher will, of course, give you proper guidance. Otherwise do the best you can. The nape of your neck should be almost straight, sloping upward towards the head. Depending on the shape of your chin, the line of the chin should be more or less straight up to the ceiling and slightly toward the feet. If you

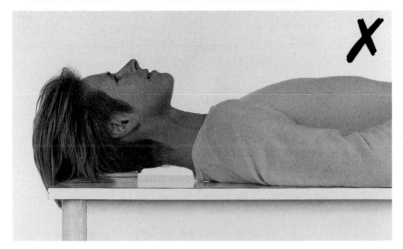

Fig. 18 *Too little head support.*

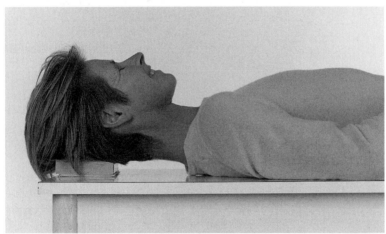

Fig. 19 *The right amount of head support.*

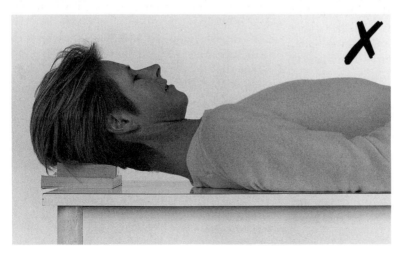

Fig. 20 *Too much head support.*

turn the following pictures sideways, you may be able to see that *Fig. 19* demonstrates the best poise of the head on the neck.

Some people require virtually no additional support for the head; others need 4–5 inches or more, depending on their height and inherited and acquired body shape. If you have a thin paperback on top, you can easily reduce the height of support after your back has flattened out further on the floor. (Some people have an uneven skull and discomfort can be avoided by making the top part of the support softer with a wad of tissues or a folded scarf.) As your back starts to change shape you will need even less head support. Most people, though, will still need some – even after years of Alexander work – because there are limits to how much an undue forward curve of the neck at the 'hump' can be reversed.

Flattening out the lower back

In order to facilitate the flattening of the back – particularly the lower back (lumbar region) – when first lying down, draw one knee towards the chest on that side of the body. Hook the fingers around the shin bone by the knee and, without forcing, pull the knee a little closer to the chest by *allowing* the shoulders and elbows to release and move apart (*Fig. 21*). Avoid tightening the arms and pulling the elbows into the sides (which will narrow the chest and shoulders). Beware of the other extreme – pushing the elbows out. There is no virtue in forcing the knee onto the chest; the mere fact of flexing the hip joints helps the lower back muscles to release. Maintain this position for a minute or two and you will notice the lower back on that side easing closer to the floor. Repeat with the other knee.

As you drew up the knees you will almost certainly have tightened your neck and pulled back your head. (And if the books are beginning to slide under the neck, move them until they are under the skull again.) Next time, remind yourself to pause before drawing up each knee. Then give the directions, with the teacher's initial help:

Let my neck release, to let my head ease out between my shoulders, to let my back lengthen and widen and flatten out on the floor.

Continue the directions as you draw up the knee. As you remember more frequently to give directions to the primary control *before and during* movement, there will be less and less interference with your coordination.

To return the leg to its position with the foot flat on the floor, think of your head easing out between your shoulders, release your fingers and let your knee describe an arc towards the ceiling as the foot and lower leg, relaxed, drop gently down onto the floor slightly wide of the hip.

After this, some 'slack' may have appeared in the lower back and the releasing muscles may need more space to lengthen further. To take out that slack – without forcing – follow this procedure. Again inhibit the immediate response to get set for the movement: leave yourself alone (non-doing). Then, give directions to the primary control. Push your heels down into the floor and let your knees point up to the ceiling, so that as your hips lift off the floor – only a fraction of an inch is necessary – they also move slightly away from the head and out towards the feet, tilting the pelvis slightly (*Fig. 22*). This tilting movement can be assisted by hands placed underneath the hips. Again let your attention be on maintaining the freedom of the neck during this movement so that you do not lose in the upper spine what you gain in length in the lower spine. This tilting movement can be repeated once or twice more as the back continues to release and lengthen during your period of lying down.

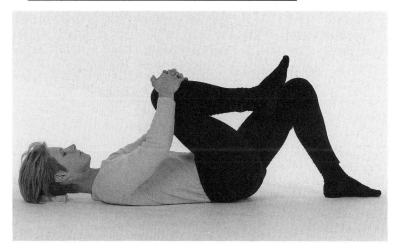

Fig. 21 Flattening out the lower back.

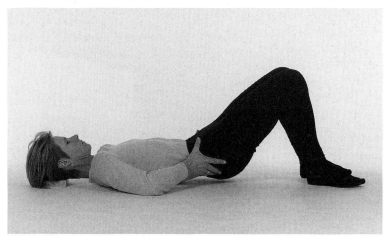

Fig. 22 Taking any 'slack' out of the lower back. Spot the deliberate mistake (neck tightening unduly to make the movement!).

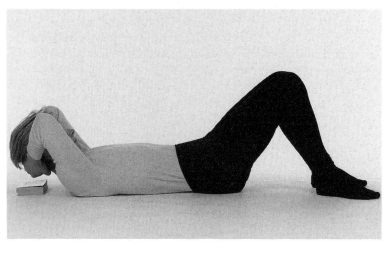

Fig. 23 Gently easing out the neck and upper back.

Easing out the middle/upper spine

To extend the stretch along the rest of the back when first lying down, leaving the neck alone, place the hands underneath the head to raise it and the upper back slightly off the floor and very gently stretch out the spine (*Fig. 23*). Remove the hands and again remind yourself to let the neck release by allowing the head to fall gently onto the books again.

Arm positions

1) Let the hands rest on the lower abdomen, fingers released and elbows out to the sides, giving space for the shoulders to release and spread out on the floor. Do not try to pull the shoulders back onto the floor (*Fig. 24*). The directions to an arm, TO BE GIVEN FOLLOWING DIRECTIONS TO THE PRIMARY CONTROL, are:

Let the shoulder release and spread sideways, to let the elbow extend out to the side, to let the hand ease out of the wrist and the fingers to lengthen out of the hand.

Repeat on the other side, after directions to the NHB relationship and then both arms at the same time. Remember not to try to 'do' these directions: think of them purely as messages from the brain to the body and allow the parts of the body concerned to respond in their own way in their own time.

2) Another arm position is to place the elbows out to the side as before, but with the wrists curving slightly inwards, forearms resting by the sides, hands and fingers on the floor and pointing towards the feet (*Fig. 25*). The directions are:

Let the shoulder release and spread sideways; continue the extension out to the elbow, to let the wrist curve inwards to the body and the fingers to lengthen out of the hand towards the feet

Repeat on the other side and then with both arms. The difficulty for many people with this position is that it highlights excessive tension in the forearm and shoulder girdle; placing a book of suitable thickness under the hand, until the arm and shoulder have released sufficiently to manage without, can make this position less uncomfortable.

3) The 'crucifix' position is to place the arms out to the sides, palms upwards. With the upper arms out but slightly down towards the feet, forearms straight out from the elbows, the widening of the back and moving apart of the shoulder blades will be facilitated; this is particularly useful if your

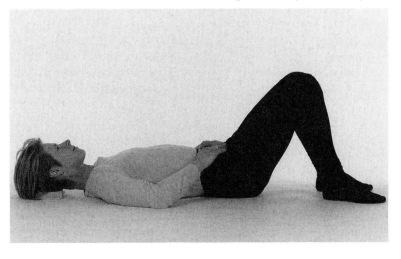

Fig. 24 Let the shoulders release and spread out on the floor.

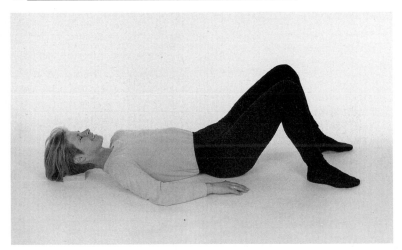

Fig. 25 Wrists curving slightly inwards, forearms resting by the sides.

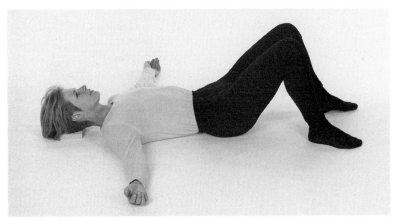

Fig. 26 The 'crucifix' position.

shoulders are very rounded (*Fig. 26*). The directions are:

Let the shoulder release and spread sideways, to let the arm lengthen out from the shoulder and the fingers to lengthen out of the hand.

With all these positions you may need – once or twice – to move the arms outwards a small distance to allow more space for the muscles of the arm and shoulders to release still further.

Leg positions
1) The main position of the legs is as described before: feet about shoulders-width apart and pointing very slightly outwards, knees aiming up towards the ceiling (*Fig. 27*). The feet should be a foot to a foot and a half's distance away from the buttocks. The weight of the leg should be evenly supported over the foot. If the knee starts to fall inwards/outwards, pressure will be localized on the inside/outside of the foot. If the legs are too relaxed, they will tend to wobble; if they are too tense, effort will be wasted in supporting the legs and the joint surfaces will be jammed together. What is required is a balanced tone in the leg and pelvic muscles where just enough work is being done to maintain the position of the legs. This will be facilitated by giving

Fig. 27 Feet about shoulders-width apart and pointing very slightly outwards.

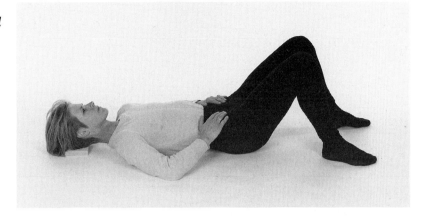

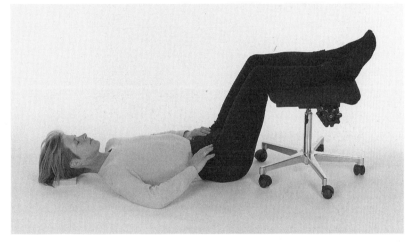

Fig. 28

directions to each leg, FOLLOWING DIRECTIONS TO THE PRIMARY CONTROL:

Let the hip release to let the knee point up out of the hip and up out of the ankle (towards the ceiling) and slightly apart from the other knee; and to let the toes lengthen out of the foot.

Repeat for the other leg and then for both legs. The effect of flexing the hip and knee joints is to tilt the pelvis slightly forwards (up to the ceiling) and it will help reduce the curve in an unduly arched (lordotic) lower back. Furthermore, although the ankles are not flexed, *this lying down releasing position allows the brain to* register *that the legs can work and yet the NHB relationship does not need to be disturbed – of great significance when we consider bending and lifting.*

2) If the lower back is acutely painful, it can be particularly helpful to support the lower legs on a low sofa or bed or chair (*Fig. 28*).

3) If you are feeling drowsy, turn the toes inwards a little and let the knees fall together so the legs won't flop (*Fig. 29*).

4) If the legs cramp or wobble excessively, spend some time with the knees supported on large cushions. (This is a little

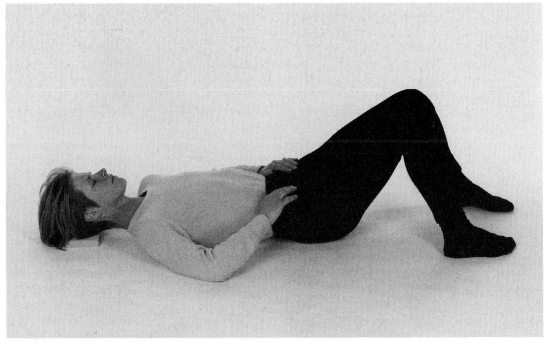

Fig. 29 Cat-napping position.

less effective in releasing the lower back, and in time you should aim to use only the main leg position.) The directions are then:

Let the legs release at the hips to allow them to lengthen out of the hips along the floor; the soles of the feet to tend away from the crown of the head, all the joint surfaces to separate away from each other.

What should I be thinking of while lying down?

Easing out the back as suggested takes a few minutes. Let the supporting surface and your directions allow further release to take place. Give several sets of directions, allowing a pause between each set to help prevent 'directing' being a 'doing'. Let your eyes remain open while giving directions. For the remaining minutes of your main lying-down period you can be quiet, listen to music or just drift off to sleep for a while if you are feeling tired!

Getting up from lying down

The usual habit is to heave straight up from a lying down position, tightening the neck and pulling the chin down towards the chest. Note the similarity to sit-up exercises – the spine is forcefully flexed and compressed and you reverse the benefits of lying down.

People with acute back pain soon learn that there is another way of getting up which minimizes the pressure on the spine (*Figs. 30–38*): rolling over onto the side is a useful *preventive* measure for us all. Remember to stop and give directions at each change in position of the sequence. When you first come to standing you may notice that you are standing quite differently at first, due to your back having become longer and wider. (From standing to lying down involves the reverse sequence of movements, of course.)

When you get out of bed in the morning, roll over onto your side as before and then let your legs dangle over the side of the bed as you push yourself up to a sitting position, head leading the movement. Now, on going to bed . . .

Choice of bed and sleeping positions

If you've ever slept on a soft, sagging bed which has given you backache, it is very tempting to go to the other extreme: a bed which is too hard and does not yield to hips and shoulders when you sleep on your side – as most of us do, most of the night. The mattress should allow your spine to remain in reasonable alignment. If you cannot tell whether that is so, ask someone to check when you are lying on it on your side, your head and neck supported on a pillow; your backbone should be in line.

As far as pillows are concerned, it all depends what position you sleep in. If you sleep on your front, you can place the pillow under your chest or omit it altogether. If you place it under your head, your head will be jammed back, giving you neck and lower back stiffness and pain. If you sleep on your back, you will probably only need a small pillow – the height of paperbacks will be a rough guide – bearing in mind you will need somewhat less as the bed will be softer than your floor support.

Sleeping on your side, you will need the support of a good quality pillow to fill in the space between your head, neck and shoulder. 'Neck' pillows, designed with a depression for the head and support for the neck, can work well if you can try them out to ensure they are of a suitable size. Otherwise, you can improvise with a folded towel inside the pillow case against the front edge of the pillow. If you sleep on your back, however, you will find that the neck pillow tends to push the neck upwards, rather than allowing it to release downwards, which is what is needed.

A sore lower back can often be improved by avoiding the twisting which tends to take place when the upper leg falls across the lower as you lie on your side. This can be done by placing a large pillow under the uppermost knee or between the knees. Discomfort in the upper spine can sometimes be alleviated by placing a pillow under the upper arm to avoid it pulling the back out of alignment. Some people assume a foetal position in bed – the spine a C-shape – which will tend to exacerbate any back problem; it is fine to have the knees bent up, of course, but the spine should be lengthened out.

Because we shift about many times in the course of the night, how can advice about ideal sleeping positions be practicable? The answer is that you can at least fall asleep in a comfortable position; and when you wake up at night, adjust your position as necessary. In time you will be able to train yourself so that you spend less time in awkward positions.

Reading in bed can be a problem in seeing the book without pushing the neck and upper back forward with large pillow(s). Two ways of dealing with this are to have the book suspended by a device above your head (*see Fig. 100*) and apart from the need to turn pages, this also avoids aching arms and cold hands! The other option is to use a large foam wedge underneath the length of the back.

We shall now see – more importantly – how the Alexander Technique can improve body use in *activity*.

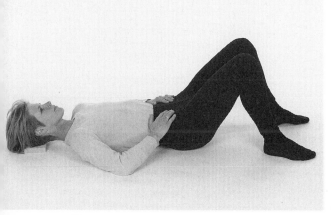

Fig. 30

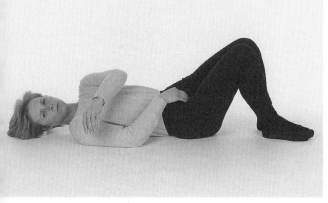

Fig. 31

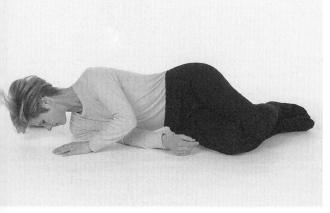

Fig. 32

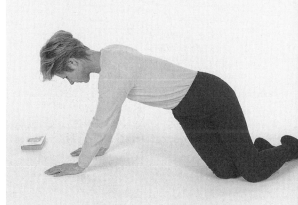

Fig. 33

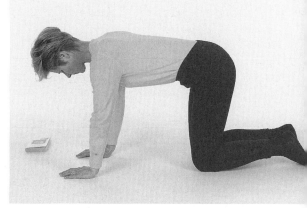

Fig. 34

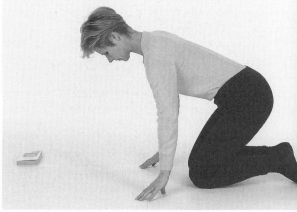

Fig. 35

Fig. 36

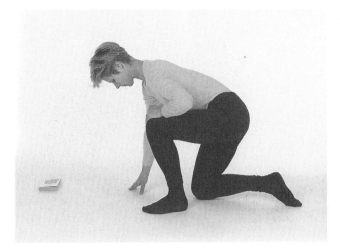

Fig. 37

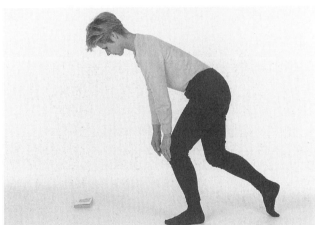

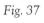

Figs. 30–38 Getting up
from lying down – avoiding
undue stiffening of the neck.

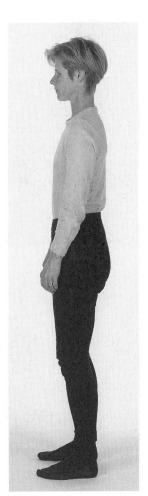

Fig. 38

CHAPTER 6

Keeping your head

Common expressions provide clues to the links between states of mind and our physical responses, for example: 'he lost his head'; 'she was always level-headed'. In this chapter we are going to look at some aspects of how we move the head in relation to the neck. This will extend your understanding of the primary control, the prerequisite for taking stock of all movement. We are also going to try to clarify the meaning of the directions used in the Alexander Technique and their relationship to each other.

Whatever the position of the head, it should be freely balanced on top of the neck. This involves probably the most important joint in the human body – the atlanto-occipital joint – where the first vertebra in the neck articulates with the base of the skull. The freedom of this joint affects not only the efficient orientation of the sense organs but also the freedom of all joints in the body.

Tilting movements of the head

Most forward and backward tilting movements of the head can and should take place *primarily* at the atlanto-occipital joint – not further down or at the base of the neck. The head tends to follow the movements of the eyes. When we look down, the head is often thrust forwards and down with the neck. Muscles at the front of the neck contract and the upper back is often humped. That is

Fig. 39 Pulling forward and down.

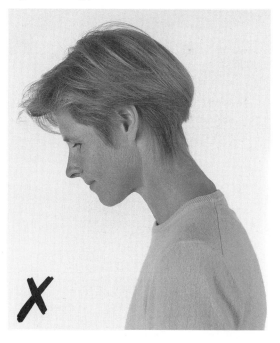

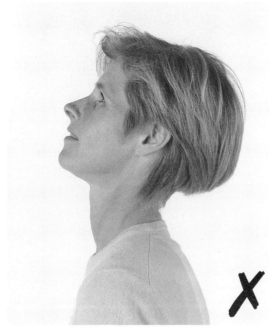

Fig. 40 Pulling back and down.

Fig. 41 'Forward and up' while looking down.

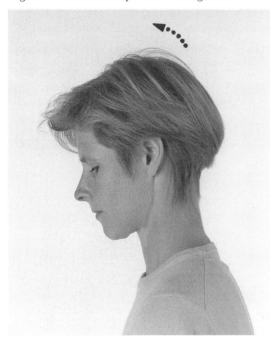

how the majority of people sit – slumped – working at a desk all day long (*Fig. 39*).

To look up, the head is usually pulled backwards and down into the shoulders by a contraction of the big muscles at the back of the neck. It is as though the head is fixed to a pole – most of the neck – so that movement of the head is initiated further down the neck (*Fig. 40*).

You can investigate this for yourself by making a nodding movement of the head with a hand placed round the back of the neck. The neck is usually 'broken' just above the seventh cervical vertebra (you can readily feel this most prominent vertebra just at the base of your neck). That is a very inefficient movement – involving contraction through the whole body – when you need to look up or down. It can produce great stiffness and discomfort at the base of the neck and top of the shoulders when driving a car or working at a desk.

Alternatively, you can make a more economical movement with the head lightly balanced *on top* of the neck. The help of a teacher will be essential to explore the subtleties of this kind of freedom of the head on the neck, but there are certain things you can understand for yourself. Wrap the hand lightly round the back of the neck as before. Pause and allow your head to nod forwards on top of the neck slowly and a small distance at a time by thinking of releasing the back of the top of the neck (*Fig. 41*). You should notice the neck staying more in contact with your hand and you may feel less downward pressure through the front of your neck and chest.

To allow the head to tilt backwards, pause and think of the front of the neck gradually releasing and lengthening to let the head roll back a little way on top of the neck – rather than pulling it backwards. Again pause and think of the head releasing very slightly forward on top of the neck – to relieve any jamming back of the head into the neck and shoulders – and you should restore a freer balance, to let the head roll back even further. You should notice less pressure on the hand at the back of the neck this time (*Fig. 42*).

Of course there are occasions when you will need more than the 10–15° of forward, and the same amount of backward, movement at the head–neck joint. If you remember to think of your neck lengthening as it releases, you will have more chance of allowing appropriate movement at *all* the joints in the neck.

Turning the head

The Alexander Technique aims to restore and maintain the freedom of the head on the neck – whatever the position of the head. To be sure, if you work in static positions for long periods, there are positions of the head which are more or less mechanically advantageous: it doesn't make any sense to keep the head a long way forward or backward or to the side – yet this is what we often do when concentrating hard.

Wild animals need to be able to move their heads quickly to orientate their sense organs to signs of impending danger. Trying to cross a busy road junction involves human beings in making similar quick turning movements of the eyes and head. Such movements, should the head pull back and down into the shoulders, will be jerky, stiff and slow (*Fig. 43*). This can be improved if you remember to pause – if only for a fraction of a second – to allow your neck to undo to let your head go forward and up. Your head should then be able to turn more freely and quickly – like a well-greased bearing – following the movement of your eyes (*Fig. 44*).

It should now be apparent why head-rolling exercises are inadvisable: they tend to

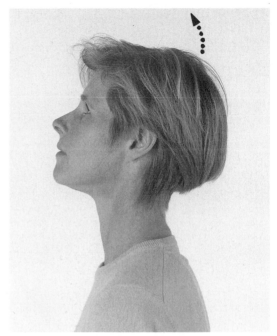

Fig. 42 'Forward and up' while looking up.

Fig. 43 Pulling back and down while turning the head.

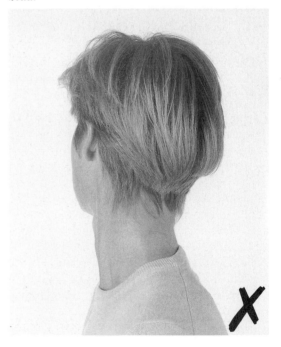

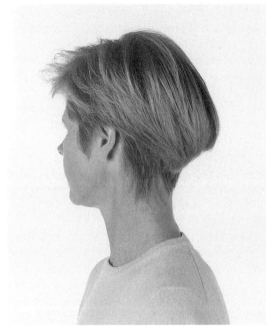

Fig. 44 Turning the head with freedom.

shift tension about, rather than release it; they blur the distinction between significantly different kinds of movement; and they may cause joints to grind and produce dizziness in those with osteoarthritic changes in their spine.

More on directions

Alexander said that the directions should be given in proper sequence and eventually all at once. But what are the directions meant to convey, and how do they work together?

Remember that first of all they are *preventive*: that is, they are given to prevent the head pulling back and down – or forward and down; and to prevent the back shortening and narrowing, thus avoiding the collapse and contraction of the whole stature. Directions are expanding tendencies *within* the body rather than actual movements of the body.

A skilled teacher's hands will give you the

actual experience of these directions; this can speak to you more than any amount of verbal explanation, although both are necessary. It will take some time before you develop a clear sense of the directions. In the early stages, if you think you can feel what they are, you are probably trying to 'do' them.

Let the neck be free, to let the head go forward and up

Macdonald describes this as an unlocking of the head on the atlanto-occipital joint so that the head, instead of being jammed back and down into the neck, *tends* forward out of the neck. The head can then move freely on the neck to any position.

The *up* direction of the head allows the neck to lengthen – very, very slightly – which then permits lengthening all the way along the rest of the spine. The resultant 'forward and up' direction is a curve rather than linear. Where precisely 'forward and up' points to varies according to the alignment of the body and its position in space. If you are upright, the direction will be almost vertical; the more you lean forwards, the more forwards it will be. (In diving, its orientation may have to change rapidly through 360 degrees!) And its orientation will change as your use improves.

To let the back lengthen and widen

'Lengthening' the back in the Alexander sense is totally different from the crude and forceful treatment of 'traction': the rack was a form of medieval torture and traction will no doubt, one day, be considered quite barbaric and harmful. The lengthening of the spine is the gentlest separation of the vertebrae away from each other so that pressure on the intervertebral discs and all the joints is reduced.

This lengthening of the spine needs to be immediately balanced by the widening of the back. This can be understood partly as a lateral widening across the whole of the back – shoulder blades releasing down and apart from each other, allowing the upper arms to rotate slightly inwards, the elbows tending to curve slightly out and forwards – and partly as a tendency for the lower back to fan out or swell out backwards so that an excessively arched or sway back is reduced (*Figs. 45 and 46*).

Directions in the Alexander Technique work in subtle *opposition* to each other, pro-

Figs. 45 and 46 The directions and how they work in relation to each other.

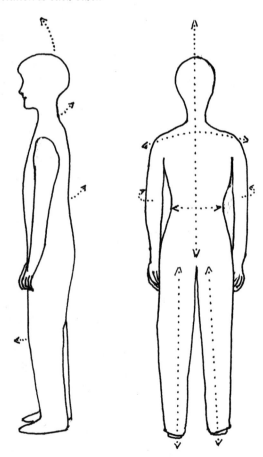

ducing at once a great sense of stability in the body and a lightness and subtle responsiveness – quite different from the heavy deadness of relaxation. The head has a forward bias in relation to the top of the neck and the rest of the spine (the whole of the spine should function as a unit). In opposition to this, the back tends backwards, and as the lower back swells out, the hips are carried backwards. If the knees unlock slightly forwards – away from the hips and lower back – the pelvis can very slightly tilt forwards, the buttocks relax and the natural dynamic balance of the whole body is restored.

Alexander used the word 'back' as a kind of shorthand, not only for the back, but also for the whole torso or trunk. You might find it helpful to conceive of the neck and torso as two cylinders, the smaller one tending to be telescoped into the larger one. As you give the directions and allow the neck to release, the smaller cylinder expands and emerges out of the bigger cylinder.

Misha Magidov's analogy is very helpful: he describes the use of the limbs subordinate to the neck, head and torso in this way: imagine the neck/torso as a kind of water tank and the limbs as hoses. As you give directions to the primary control you build up a head of pressure in the water tank and water can then flow out through the limbs as you progressively release the joints. Directions flow from the centre outwards.

Use of the eyes and states of mind

Beware of rolling your eyes upwards as you send directions! This usually happens when the directions are being forced. It produces the opposite of what is required: the chin will be raised, the neck tightened and the head pulled back and down.

Concentration is a state of mind which

tends to produce tension and stiffening of the body. What the Alexander Technique aims to cultivate is a kind of scanning awareness where what is focused on at a given moment – the 'figure' – does not lose its 'ground'. This 'expanded field of attention' (as Frank Pierce Jones called it[1]) therefore contains – as well as the usual sensory information and thoughts and emotions – a rich kinaesthetic awareness. An alert, calm state of mind has its corresponding physical counterpart. In relation to vision, the brows will not be knitted and the eyes will be free to move according to interest; not glazed or fixed or staring but blinking regularly and easily. (Psychologists use the blink rate as a measure of attention: if a subject is concentrating hard, blinking almost stops; if they become anxious and over-stimulated, it is very rapid.)

There is an approach to the re-education of the use of the eyes called the *Bates method* which overlaps to a small degree with Alexander's work. W.H. Bates was an ophthalmologist who claimed that many people did not need stronger and stronger glasses for refractive errors; they could be retrained to see more efficiently so that they did not need to use glasses at all. It seems to me there is much in this approach to help anyone with certain sorts of eye problems – at least as much for the self-knowledge it can bring. I do believe though, as Aldous Huxley did, that you need the Alexander Technique as a basis from which to make specific improvements.[2] Myopia in my right eye that developed in adolescence improved dramatically during my Alexander training without any specific work on seeing. I also had a very convincing demonstration from a teacher of the Bates method that when I became anxious about not being able to make out the smallest letters on the eye chart, my vision became more blurred. I did find, however, that giving directions to the NHB relationship was the most effective way of letting the letters come into focus.

Movement of the eyes in relation to the head

As you begin releasing your neck so that your head is less pulled back, you may notice that your eye level tends to drop slightly below horizontal. This happens because movement of the eyes tends to be bound up with the movement of the head.

The horizontal gaze is usually associated with the fixing backwards of the head on the neck (you very slightly look down your nose!). But if you lower your eyes to try to avoid your head being pulled back, be careful not to over-compensate and pull the chin down! Instead, allow your eyes to move more often independently of the head. We do not exploit this possibility enough: the eyes can be allowed to move when small shifts of glance are required, rather than having to employ the bigger neck muscles to move the weighty head. At the same time, take care not to lock the head on the neck to force the eyes to move! This new use of the eyes in relation to the head will feel strange at first.

Eye movement is very much bound up with our sense of balance. One theory on the causes of misuse is that, as hunter-gatherers for most of our evolutionary past, we would have needed to scan the terrain immediately in front of us. The slightly tilting forward of the head would have led to a neutral position of the organs of balance in the inner ear.

In the next chapter we are going to examine standing and walking. You will be learning about the need to lose a fixed, precarious balance to find a released, poised balance.

CHAPTER 7

Legging it!

People with painful backs often experience additional discomfort when having to stand for long periods. It has been suggested that Homo sapiens have not sufficiently evolved for two-legged movement – is this, at least partly, why there is such a high incidence of back pain? Tinbergen[1] thought that this was unlikely because we have had five million years to acquire the basic mechanism. His view, largely in accord with Alexander's, was that excessive sitting – many people spend as much as 24 hours in a week in front of a TV set – and the stresses of the rapid changes of modern living, are major causes.

What has been acquired – rather than genetically caused – can be undone. This is borne out by Alexander's experience and that of the teachers who followed him, and their pupils: substantial improvements in body use can be made once the principles of the Technique are grasped and properly applied.

Standing

What commonly happens when standing is that we partially collapse and then tighten to hold ourselves up. There are many different ways of standing, but a very common one

nowadays is for the lower back to be swayed, the knees locked, the hips pushed forward and body weight is centred over the heels (*Figs. 47 and 48*). This kind of misuse is exaggerated with any kind of heel to the shoe. In time, muscles at the back of the leg and the Achilles tendon (at the back of the ankle) shorten so that ankle flexibility is considerably reduced and bending movements become more and more impaired. Exercises of the toe-touching sort tend to accentuate the rigidity of the lower limbs – a form of misuse we could well do without.

Stand before a full-length mirror without clothes on and carefully observe yourself front, sides and back (you will need a second mirror – a small hand mirror will do). You will almost certainly see that you are not standing entirely straight, yet you will probably feel that you are. If your habitual stance is to sway backwards you will feel as though you are tipping forwards if you alter your alignment to a more vertical one. This is one problem in trying to correct postural defects. The other problem, and a more serious one in trying to make such a change directly by yourself, is that of trying to hold what you think is the 'correct' posture (*Fig. 49*).

What is needed, of course, is a way of

standing that allows freedom of movement with little effort. When the knees are locked, other joints tend to fix and your balance will be tied to that position. Suppose you are travelling on crowded public transport and you have to stand. The constant movement will tend to push you off balance. In such a situation, the temptation is to brace even more to resist falling over. Standing up then involves an inordinate amount of muscular work. However, if you let your knees release a little so that your feet can 'ground' as you ease upwards out of the hips – like a child's weighted toy that always falls upright – you

can discover an unstable equilibrium where you will be able to sway easily with the train's movement without fear of falling over. (Even without the challenge of some external force acting on you, you can get the idea of this by moving gently, while lengthening, forward and backward and from side to side on the spot with and without knees locked.)

Released standing

Now let's look in some detail at how to improve standing. You can stand with feet fairly close together and side by side or with one slightly behind the other.

Figs. 47 below and 48 below right The common sway-back.

Fig. 49 Over-tense standing.

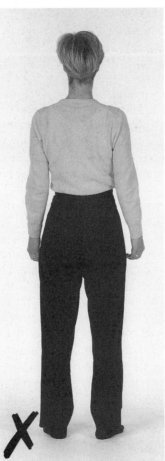

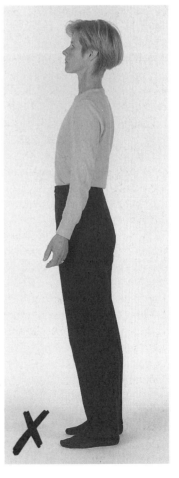

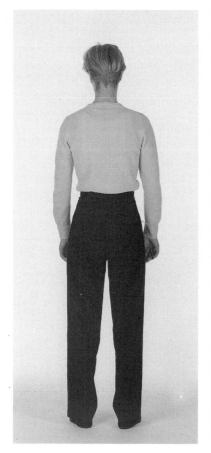 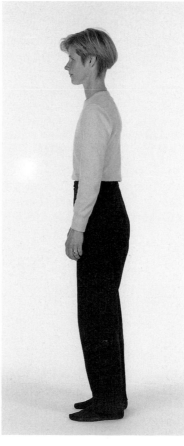

Figs. 50 far left and 51 left Released standing, feet side-by side: a longer, wider back; the palms tend to face backwards.

Fig. 52 right Released standing, feet one behind the other.

Feet side by side and apart. The farther apart the feet are placed, the more the toes should be pointed outwards. (Should you bend your knees, they could then hinge in the direction the feet are pointing.) Many people, though, stand with feet turned outwards even when they are quite close together. (This is usually accompanied by a tendency in classical ballet to unduly narrow the lower back.) If you change your usual splayed-feet position so that the toes point only very slightly outwards when the feet are close together, it will probably feel at first as though you are pigeon-toed – yet another classic illustration of faulty sensory appreciation!

Remind yourself not to try to 'do' the directions, but think them: let the neck be free to let the head go forward and up, to let the back lengthen and widen. Check you are not holding your breath or fixing your gaze. While continuing the idea of lengthening, let the lower back widen – that is, to swell out backwards. (You might find it helpful to think of your back 'smiling'.) As you think up out of your hips, allowing your back to widen, there should be a tendency for the hips to ease slightly backwards. At the same time let your knees release slightly forwards to counterbalance the whole back tending backwards, while continuing to think of lengthening along your spine. Your weight should be centred over the arches of your feet, that is, in a balanced way over the whole of the feet (*Figs. 50 and 51*).

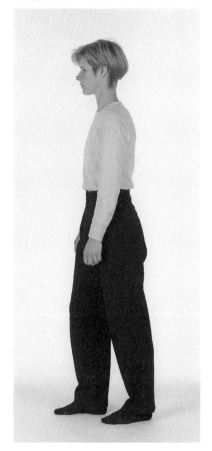

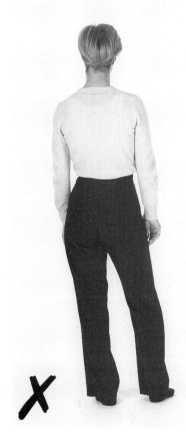

Fig. 53 Leaning on one hip: back twisted and collapsing.

Feet one slightly behind the other and apart. An alternative stance – and, of course, there are any number of permutations – is to place one foot slightly in advance of the other (*Fig. 52*). The legs provide a firm base of support, to prevent the hip sagging to the side and to avoid the lower back twisting and compressing – a common adolescent pose (*Fig. 53*).

You can, of course, alternate the legs. An exception would be if one leg is longer than the other – as it may be in someone who has broken a leg. It may then be preferable to allow the longer leg to bend a little more than the other – and that leg should be placed forwards. This will tend to reduce the tilting up of the hip on that side and the twisting of the lower back.[2]

Walking

Walking is widely regarded as one of the most beneficial forms of exercise for people of all ages. Most parts of the body are involved and it gently challenges the cardio-vascular system. You can go at your own pace and it needs no special time set aside for it, although you may want to do so. Some people enjoy the opportunity for quiet reflection; and others appreciate the obser-vation of their surroundings or conversation with a companion.

The experience of walking for its own sake can also be a great pleasure. What a marvellous instrument the human body is when moving easily, freely, gracefully!

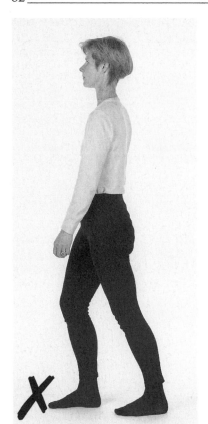 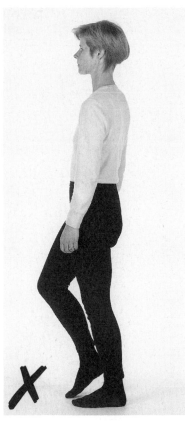

Figs. 54 and 55 How not to walk: falling down onto the front leg compresses all the joints; notice how the leg leads and the back sways.

We began to walk at about the age of one and yet we do not know *how* we walk. Back pain, following an accident or injury or pregnancy, may force us to think for the first time about the mechanics of walking. How much better to understand how we should coordinate ourselves so that problems might be prevented.

Walking: falling down or falling up?

If you ask anyone how it is that they walk – what is involved in the movement – there is usually a long silence. The reply finally comes 'Well, of course, I put one leg in front of the other.' If the question is then asked, 'What about the rest of you?' there is usually a total blank!

The commonest error in walking is to let the legs dictate the movement, without regard to the rest of the body. The swinging forwards of the leg is associated with a tendency to lift one hip up and forwards; and to sway back and slightly twist the lower back to maintain balance. The lower leg is often kicked forward, ankle stiff and toes curled back; and the heel crashes heavily down on the floor as the head and neck move forwards and *down*, compressing all the joints in the body (*Figs. 54 and 55*). As the foot hardly clears the ground, tripping over unseen objects is common, and on uneven ground balance is precarious.

Figs. 56 far right and 57 right Improved walking: the head leads, the body follows, then the leg.

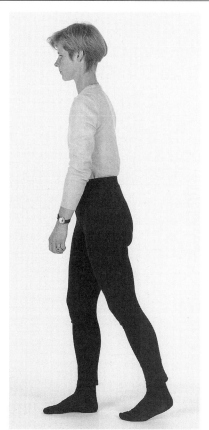 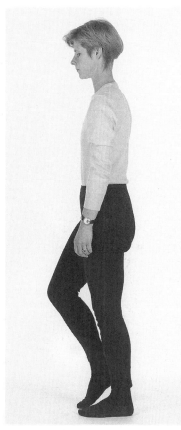

Instead of falling down onto one leg after the other, we should aim to fall upwards! *The head should lead forwards and up, the body should follow and finally the appropriate leg should move forward to support the body. (Figs. 56 and 57).*

Walking: the first step

1) Stand just behind and between two dining chairs, their backs towards you, in front of a mirror (only one chair is shown in the photographs). Lightly take hold of the backs of the chairs, fingers pointing straight down to the floor, elbow tending outwards. (Having understood more about the use of the arms – chapters 8 and 9 – you might want to return to this procedure.) The point of the chairs is to assist in the early stages so

that if you lose your balance you do not need to stiffen to regain it. Your feet should be a few inches apart and not splayed out.

Give directions and continue to think of lengthening upwards keeping balanced over both feet. Check to make sure you are not grabbing onto the chair-backs. While continuing to lengthen, raise one knee in order to lift all the foot off the floor except the toes. You may notice at first that the hip lifts up and thrusts forwards a little, accompanied by an arching of the lower back. If your knee turns slightly inwards or outwards then the weight on the foot tends more towards the big toe or the little toe (*Figs. 58 and 59*).

How should you go about changing this unnecessary movement? It is important to

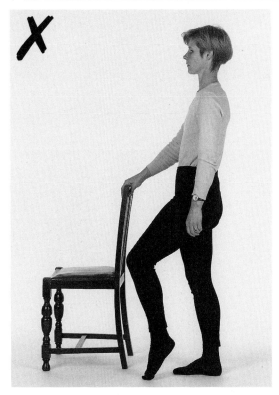

Fig. 58

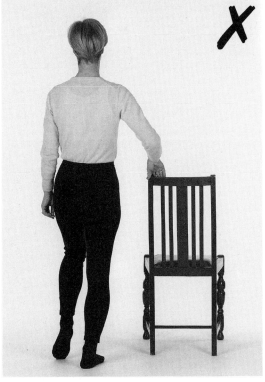

Fig. 59

realize that you should only try to change it indirectly by working with the process by which you can achieve your end. If you try to do the movement 'correctly', you will almost certainly stiffen. Your primary intention should be to allow your neck to be free, to allow your head to go forward and up to maintain the length and width of your torso; secondarily, and while directing the NHB relationship, allow your knee to lift itself in a forward direction away from your hip and lower back (which should remain back). You may not find this easy at first; but if you patiently stick to the 'means-whereby' – aided by a teacher – you will find your walking will improve and continue to improve when you are on your own (*Figs. 60 and 61*).

It is then a question of refining the coordi-

nation. See how slowly and smoothly you can allow the movement to do itself. Remember not to hold your breath or tighten your arms. Avoid looking down at your legs because you'll probably want to pull down: use a mirror instead to observe what is happening. Repeat with the other leg.

2) Next you can raise the knees alternately as if walking on the spot. Don't rush this either; if you attend to the primary control each time you lift the knee *and* as you let the heel come down onto the floor, you will maintain length and minimize hip sway.

3) The last stage is to allow your head to move forward and up and – as the body follows – let the knee lift away from the hip and lower back to peel the foot completely

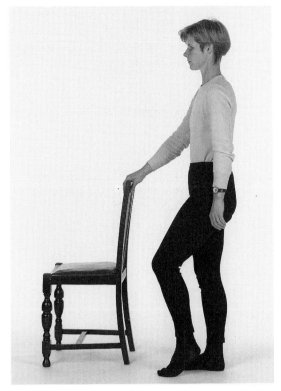

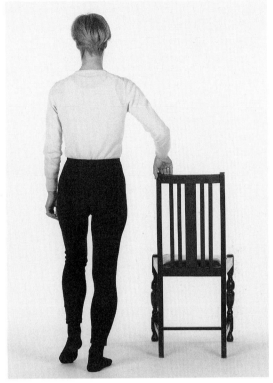

Fig. 60

Fig. 61

off the floor. Allow the ankle, foot and toes to remain 'loose' and the foot will come softly down on the floor as you lengthen along the spine to take your first step; avoid bracing the knee. You are now walking! If you managed to prevent the arching of your lower back, the heel will probably contact the floor just before the rest of the foot.

When walking, you will probably find you need to take slightly shorter strides than usual – especially at first – to make it easier to maintain the NHB relationship. It can be helpful when walking any distance to stop and stand still from time to time to observe what has been happening. The more you end-gain, the more you will distort your lower back. Renew your directions to undo the pulling down and sway-back. You will then be able to maintain a more expanded quality of

movement for longer periods of time. Eventually you will be able to extend your stride and not lose your poise (see picture of Alexander walking, page 17).

While directing the NHB relationship, let the shoulders release and spread sideways and the arms should swing slightly and easily to the movement of the body: each arm will move forward with its opposite leg (contra-lateral movement).

T'ai Chi slow walking

Slow-motion T'ai Chi walking can help improve normal walking and walking on stairs or on sloping ground. In this procedure, let the foot come softly down *before* moving the head in a forwards and up direction to transfer the weight slowly onto the front leg. As you lift the knee, be careful not to arch your lower back. You can also try walking backwards very slowly, letting as much as possible of the back part of the foot make contact with the floor before shifting the weight onto it. Initially, if you take small steps backwards, you will find it much easier. The basic idea is to remain 'single-weighted' until the moment you decide to transfer your weight to the other leg: that is, the foot you have moved (the leg stays 'empty') could be moved back or to somewhere else, before committing any weight to it.

Standing on tiptoes

The temptation here is to swing the weight forward on to the front part of the feet by raising the chest (*Fig. 62*). The consequent hollowing of the lower back is often accentuated by the need to look up and to raise the arms at the same time; as in hanging washing on a line or reaching up to a shelf.

To experience the back staying back while rising on the toes, stand with your heels close to a relatively smooth wall or door. Give directions to the primary control letting the back gently flatten as much as it can against the wall while lengthening upwards. Renew directions and letting your head lead, allow your back to slide up the wall as you slowly rise onto the balls of your feet and then onto your toes (*Figs. 63 and 64*). Stop for a moment and then think of your head releasing forwards and up as you let your ankles relax to return to standing.

Fig. 62   *Fig. 63*   *Fig. 64*   *Fig. 65*

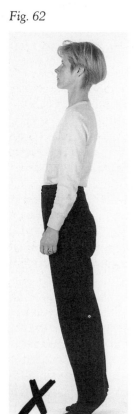
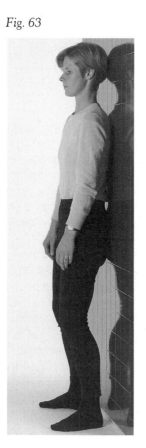
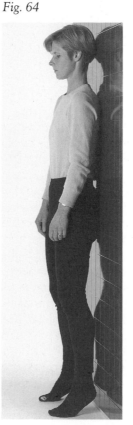
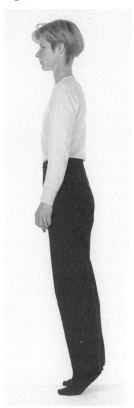

Next, let yourself lengthen – inclining slightly forwards on your ankles to let your weight shift over the balls of your feet – and your back will come away from the surface behind you. Without the wall actually there to remind you to keep your back back, *think* your back back against an imaginary wall as you let your head lead you up onto your toes (*Fig. 65*).

Walking up and down stairs

Walking upstairs usually involves lurching onto the front leg and then retracting the head as the back leg is swung through. Walking downstairs involves falling down onto the front leg. In both cases, body weight is transferred prematurely onto the front leg – accompanied by a pulling down (*Figs. 66 and 67*). T'ai Chi concepts again provide insights into what is required: the idea of remaining single-weighted and 'rooted' in one leg, the other leg being 'empty', until it is able to 'root'.

To see how this applies in walking upstairs, begin in a standing position, both feet on one step and give directions. Continue lengthening while balancing on one leg (single-weighted, rooted), lift the other knee away from the lower back and hip and let the foot come softly down (this leg remains 'empty'). Then let the head lead forward and up, body following, as the back leg thrusts down to transfer the weight to the front leg. (The back leg thrust begins at the heel and then carries on through to the ball of the foot.) (*Fig. 68*).

As you continue walking upstairs the sequence of movement is: head leads, body follows, back foot thrusts down, front knee is lifted up, foot softly comes down, weight transfers to front leg. To help get the idea of not transferring the weight onto the front leg prematurely, you can occasionally practise the first step up, as before: that is, balancing on one leg, lifting the other knee up and

letting the foot come softly down. Pause before transferring the weight to the front leg.

To go downstairs, balance on one leg, and as that knee bends lift the other knee up and let the foot come softly down. Then transfer the weight to it. You will be aware of the back leg needing to bend more and work harder than usual (*Fig. 69*). This will prevent the usual jarring of the joints and the tightening of the neck and back. The continuous movement of flexing and extending your knees will stop your thigh muscles seizing up! Always remember the primary directions.

To allow the whole of the foot to make contact on narrow stairs, in order to help the leg thrust and to avoid slipping, try negotiating stairs at an angle of about 45°.

Running and jogging

Running is difficult to improve unless you have had a substantial number of Alexander lessons. The first movement commonly made by most runners is to pull the head down; and this pulling down tends to get worse the longer you run, producing excessive joint pressure and muscular tension. You only have to observe the strain on their faces and the lack of ease of many joggers to wonder if they are doing themselves more harm than good!

On the contrary, if you know how to let the head lead forward and up, running becomes lighter and freer. You will notice only the smallest movement of the head up and down and from side to side as you run. Shoulders should be directed to release and spread sideways, arms moving freely, contralaterally with the legs.

Use of the arms: first considerations

In the next two chapters, use of the arms will be considered in depth. To begin thinking

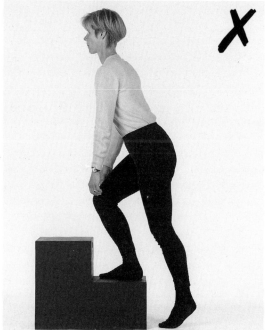 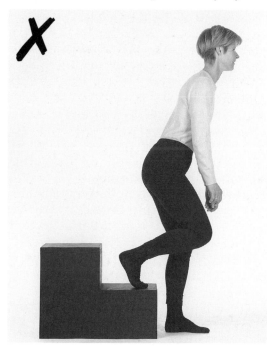

Fig. 66

Fig. 67

Fig. 68

Fig. 69

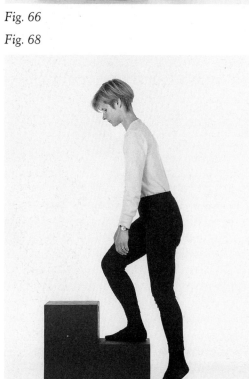 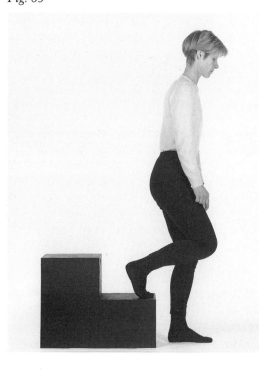

about how the use of the arms should be integrated with the rest of the body, stand sideways on to a mirror, arms at your sides. Raise the arms straight out in front to shoulder level and then higher. Notice how your back tends to sway and your hips push forward (*Fig. 70*).

This time stand with your back against a wall or door. While thinking of your back staying back and lengthening, let your shoulders release sideways from each other to let the extension continue out to the elbows and allow your hands to raise themselves slowly away from your back, which should stay as close to the wall as possible. You should notice that your shoulders do less work than they did previously (*Fig. 71*). Repeat away from the supporting surface and think of your back lengthening and tending back against an imaginary wall behind you. If you stand with your feet – one slightly behind the other as described previously – you will find it easier to let your back stay back (*Figs. 72 and 73*).

Fig. 70 right

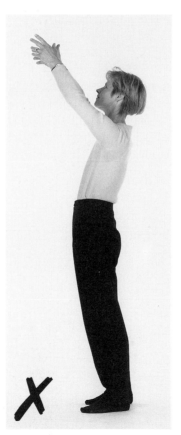
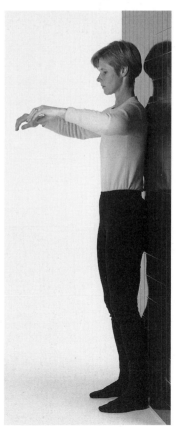

Fig. 71 far right

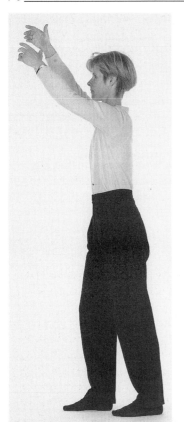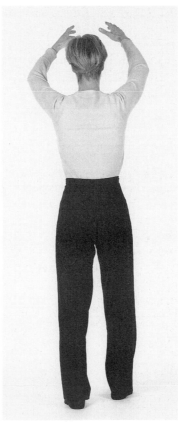

*Figs. 72 and 73 Back
lengthening and widening while
raising arms.*

Fig. 73 left

CHAPTER 8

Your ischial tuberosities

Sitting puts one-third more pressure on the spine than standing. Alexander believed that the collapsed way in which people sit for much of the day contributes greatly to the stress-related diseases and mechanical disorders so common in modern civilization.

Discovering your sitting bones (ischial tuberosities!)

In the previous chapter on standing we looked at the value of centring your body weight over the feet arches. Similarly, when sitting, if you centre your weight mainly over your sitting bones and a little over your feet, it will help you maintain a more released, upright posture.

To be clear about where your sitting bones are, sit on your hands on a reasonably level chair. Depending on your degree of padding, you will feel two knobbly parts of the pelvis, which are your sitting bones. If you make excessive effort to sit upright, notice how your weight tends to shift forward onto the thigh bones as your lower back arches (*Fig. 74*). If you slump, your weight will tend to shift onto the back part of the pelvis, which will tilt too far backwards (*Fig. 75*). Centering your body weight over

your sitting bones, then, will help towards a more expanded body use when sitting (*Fig. 76*).

Notice that if you cross one leg over the thigh of the other, your body weight tends to shift onto one sitting bone. This is accompanied by a tilting of the pelvis and twisting of the lower back (*Fig. 77*). Most people will slump with their legs crossed. If you place your hand round your waist at the back, you will be able to feel your back becoming more rounded. The third reason to avoid crossing the legs is that you interfere with blood flow, a factor in the development of varicose veins. Of course, if you usually cross your legs when you sit, it will feel uncomfortable, unnatural and awkward – at first – to change.

If it is preferable to avoid crossing your legs, what can you do with them?! Observe the amount of tension in the inner thighs and hips if you clamp your legs together. Now let them go; your knees will release forwards and slightly apart from each other. Move your feet under your knees and you will have a sensible position for your legs when sitting. Sometimes, however, there is so much residual tension in the legs that the knees still pull together. In that case you will need to keep directing them out over your

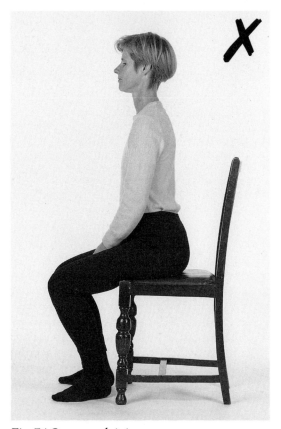

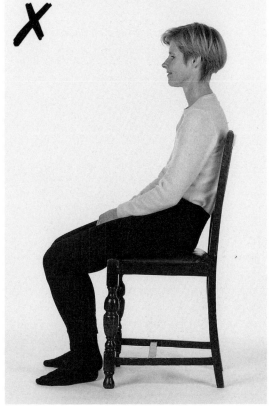

Fig. 74 Over-tensed sitting.

Fig. 75 Slumped sitting.

feet for some time until the new pattern is established. You may have difficulties with this if you wear short, tight skirts! Another possibility is to cross the legs at the ankles.

Sitting at ease

Sit as far back in the chair as you can to utilize the support provided by the back of the chair along your back. This is where many armchairs, sofas and conference chairs fail. The base is usually too long for anyone except giants: if you sit right back, your legs stick out at a ridiculous angle, often with pressure under the backs of the thighs just behind the knees; and if you sit

far enough forward to get your feet on the floor, your lower back sags badly.

Schools and other institutions are negligent in buying plastic chairs designed for *stacking* rather than for seating human beings: the back of the chair is so unstable that you need to thrust your neck forwards to stop yourself toppling backwards. Some train and coach seats also offend by a C-shaped back which pushes the back into a rounded shape, agonizing for long journeys.

When buying a chair, it is best to sit for some time in the one you are intending to buy. What feels comfortable may not prove in the long run to be the best for your back. Look for a chair with a relatively short base and a long, slightly inclined back.

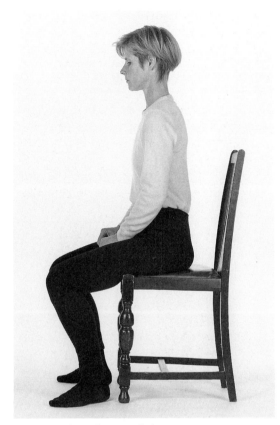

Fig. 76 Released, expanded sitting.

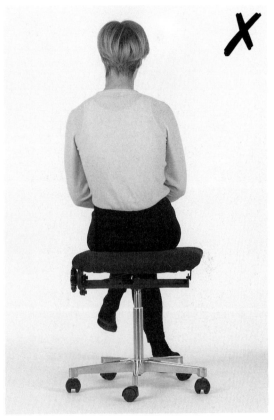

Fig. 77 Crossing the legs tends to collapse and twist the lower back.

The chair should be shaped sufficiently to prevent the lower spine collapsing, yet not force an excessive lumbar curve. The upper chair back should be straight and not shaped. Because we are all different, the same chair will not necessarily suit everyone.

Ideally, an easy chair will also have some facility for a variable degree of reclining. Beware of reclining chairs which push the neck and upper back forwards in relation to the rest of the back. When watching TV, place the screen so that you don't have to move your head and neck forwards to the screen, but that the screen effectively 'comes to you'.

Working chairs

There are two main problems of body mechanics in sitting at work. The first is the relatively static position which encourages muscles to seize up and fatigue quickly, leading to progressively more pulling downwards in sedentary workers as the day wears on; the second is the need to be close enough to your work – many people slump forwards as a consequence (Fig. 78).

Children – and some adults – tend to tip chairs forwards on their front legs so that, instead of slumping down, the whole body is inclined forwards from the hips (Fig. 79). This practice is discouraged because of stress to the chair and because it is unstable.

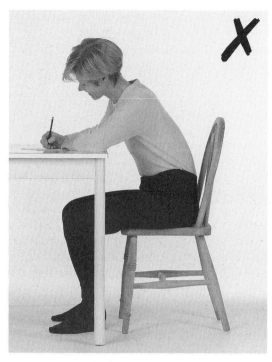

Fig. 78 Usual slumped working position.

However, the important lesson to be learnt here is that a working chair needs to be adjustable not only so that it can be raised and lowered, but also so that it is capable of being *tilted forwards*. In Victorian times, working chairs were level or tilted forwards – not tilting backwards like most modern chairs.

Vary your position as you work at your desk, which will help reduce muscle fatigue. As you give directions to the NHB relationship, muscles in the back are encouraged to lengthen. If you have been used to slumping at your desk, it will take a little while to re-

Fig. 79 Tilting the chair on its front legs points to the answer but is not the solution!

Fig. 80 A chair can be made to 'tilt' by the use of a wedge-shaped cushion.

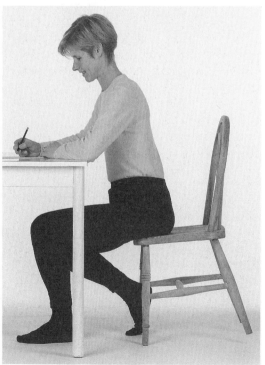

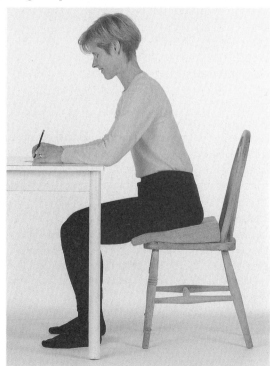

educate your back muscles to support you as they should. At first you may ache a little as your back gets used to working more as it should, so increase the amount of time you sit in the new way *gradually*.

Sit close to the front of the seat and let the head, neck and torso hinge as a unit very slightly forwards from the hips. The chair should be high enough – approaching one-third of your height – so that the angle between thigh and torso is greater than 90 degrees to help avoid rounding the lower back (see Appendix I). The slightest lumbar curve should be preserved. It should not be necessary for the neck to be poked forwards to get the eyes close enough to your work.

Available at the top end of the market is an office chair which automatically and imperceptibly moves through a tiny range of tilt as you sit, greatly reducing fatigue – invaluable for someone with severe back problems. At a very reasonable price is a 'simple working chair' (without back support – not absolutely essential in a working chair) with adjustable tilt. It is now also possible to purchase a VDU operator's chair with adjustable forward tilt and a back rest which can be moved sufficiently far forwards to provide support during a long working day (see appendix II). If your present chair does not tilt, you can improvise by putting a stout cushion under the sitting bones or, better still, have a wedge-shaped cushion made (*Fig. 80*). (see Appendix I).

Chairs are available which support the knees as well as the sitting bones. They can be an improvement on a chair whose base slopes backwards but there are three distinct problems with them and I don't think they are such a great improvement as they might appear. First of all – unless you buy the most expensive ones – you cannot raise the whole seat up and down. Secondly, as you lean forward to work, pressure tends to go onto the knees and the thighs jam into the hip

joints. Finally, in a busy office, it is tedious to have to keep moving the legs in and out from underneath you to get up. At very low cost – as suggested – you can substantially improve a badly-designed chair until you are ready to invest in a tilting chair which will enable you to plant your feet on the ground.

Hands on the chair-rail procedure

Shortly we shall be looking at the use of the arms in relation to operating a keyboard of some kind and in relation to handwriting. In his second book, Alexander described in detail a procedure in which the hands are placed on the top rail of a chair.[1] *You will need the assistance of a teacher to introduce this procedure properly to you.* It has important implications for teachers of the Alexander Technique and for all of us in using our arms in a more effective and efficient way in our daily activities. This procedure also encourages the widening of the back, and an expanded torso facilitates breathing.

Take a level chair and place a good-sized cushion at your back to allow your torso to lengthen and widen against it; place a second chair, the rail facing you, just in between your feet. Get your sitting bones as far back in the first chair as you can so that the lower back does not collapse.

1) Let the back of the hands rest on the lap, palms facing upwards. In a while you may place the hands on top of the chair-rail. First, though, inhibit your immediate desire to move the arms and allow yourself to wait and do nothing in this position. Give directions to the primary control letting your back lengthen and flatten out more against the cushion behind you. Then give secondary directions:

Let my knees tend forwards away from the hips and lower back and slightly apart from each other out over the feet. (Note the similarity to the resting position.)

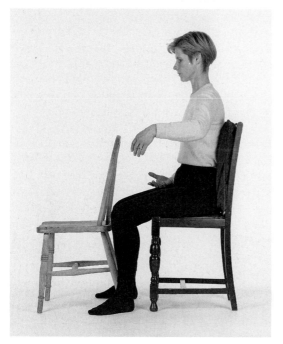

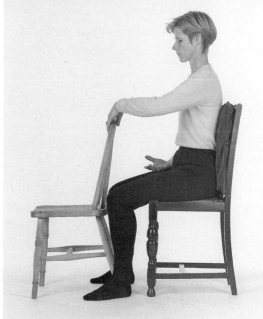

Fig. 81

Fig. 82

Fig. 83

Fig. 84

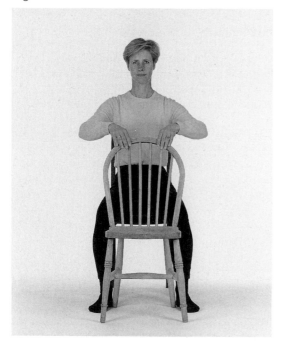

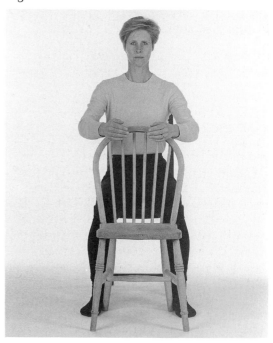

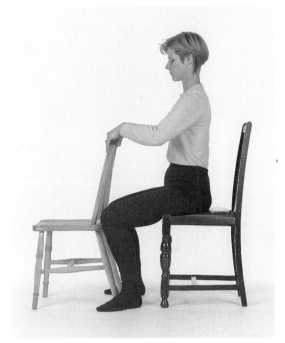

Fig. 85

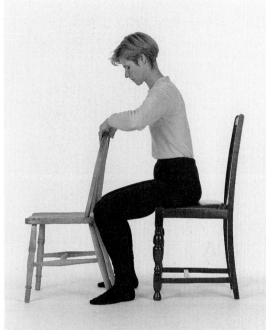

Fig. 86

Repeat the primary directions and then follow with secondary directions to the arms, in turn:

Let the shoulder release and spread sideways to continue the extension out to the elbow, to let the hand release away from the wrist and the fingers to lengthen out of the hand; that is, all the joint surfaces in the arm are directed to separate away from each other.

2) Then renew the directions to the NHB relationship, and while leaving the neck alone, lift the hand away from the torso (back staying back against the back of the chair), elbow curving sideways and forwards, to gently but firmly take hold of the top rail of the chair. The fingers should be straight (lengthening, not rigid), pointing down to the floor, letting the wrist curve slightly inwards in opposition to the elbow curving sideways (*Figs. 81 and 82*).

Again repeat the primary directions and,

while doing so, let the fingers let go of the chair-rail to let the hand return to the upper thigh once more. Repeat with the other arm.

3) Now take hold of the rail of the chair as before but with both hands. Gently lift the back of the chair up and away from you so that the back legs are fractionally off the floor. At the same time pull the elbows slightly apart and down to widen the shoulders and then let the chair rest back on the floor. Next, let the elbows drop slightly to relieve any extra work still being done by the arms.

4) Give the primary directions and then secondary directions to the arms once more to widen the shoulders and to let the elbows curve outward. In this procedure, the arms are helping both to support and widen the torso. At the same time the proper use of the primary control is helping to support the arms. Of course the arms and shoulders are

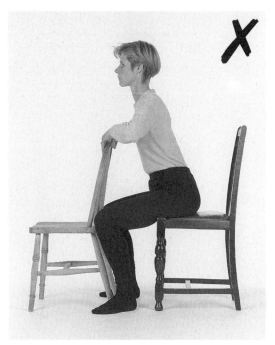

Fig. 87

joints (*Fig. 85 and 86*). Avoid collapsing the torso and pulling the shoulders and head back (*Fig. 87*). This kind of movement at the hips is needed to lean forwards to eat at the meal table, for instance.

It should now be clear why the injunction 'pull your shoulders back' is quite wrong, for it does not deal with the mechanical cause – the humped upper back – which produces the rounding of the shoulders (*Fig. 88*). And it is harmful because the attempt to pull the shoulders back causes rigidity, fixing the upper arms into the shoulder sockets and forcing the shoulder blades together. It is accompanied by a tendency to stiffen the neck, raise the chest and hollow the lower back – a military-style posture (*Fig. 89*).

The way to improve round shoulders is, therefore, to understand and remedy the general misuse out of which this particular aspect of misuse has developed (*Fig. 90*).

doing work in this position: the arms should neither be heavy nor tense. *This position of the arms is demanding but this kind of coordination is required by a string player in the bowing arm.* Do not leave the arms in this position for more than a few seconds at a time on your own, because you will tend to fix your arms and shoulders (*Fig. 83*).

A variation of hand position is to rest the heels of the hands on the chair-rail (give directions to the arms as in the lying down releasing position, when they are resting on your lower abdomen). Lightness and freedom in the use of your arms will develop as you learn to leave your neck alone (*Fig. 84*).

5) Later on, try this procedure sitting at the front of the chair. Then, to lean forwards, gently pull your elbows apart and down and let your shoulders widen further. Let the head curve in a forward and up arc to allow the torso to incline forwards from the hip

Fig. 88

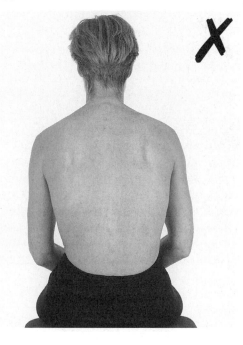

Keyboarding

We can now consider the special problems of working at a keyboard – whether typewriter, computer keyboard or piano and keyboard musical instruments. It is often quite possible to achieve the best ergonomic arrangement for using a computer. As a general rule you should be sitting high enough for the wrists to be level with, or lower than, the elbows. If the keyboard is too high – often the case with a shorter person – the shoulders will tend to hunch. The remedy is to raise the chair and utilize a foot rest. If the keyboard is too low, the wrists will flex excessively (*Fig. 91*). Either extreme can predispose you to the development of upper-limb disorders or RSI.

The next factor to consider is the positioning of the monitor. You should aim to place the screen in such a position that the information on the screen 'comes to you',

rather than you needing to squint at the screen. This requires the screen to be slanted a little upwards so that it is perpendicular to the eyes and the centre of the screen should be slightly below horizontal eye-level (*Fig. 92*). (Remember to keep moving the data close to the centre of the screen as much as possible.) Again, you can improvise if the monitor is not adjustable by using, for example, box files and folded magazines placed underneath it.

It is important to sit square on to the keyboard and monitor. Many people work at a cramped desk where the computer is to one side and they twist awkwardly from side to side. Another important aid is the use of a copyholder so that any text you need to refer to while keyboarding can be scanned by the eyes instead of having to move the head a large distance.

Computer operators need to take frequent breaks. Get up and walk around at

Fig. 89

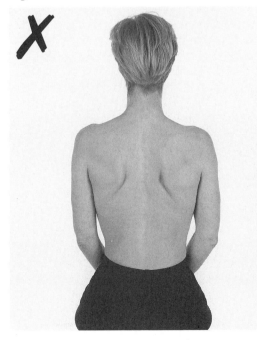

Fig. 90

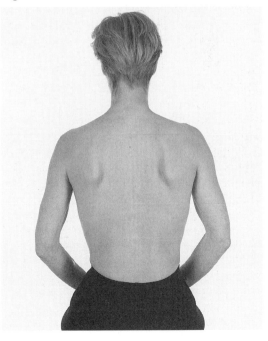

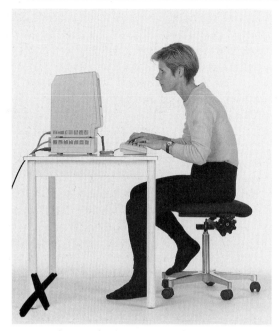

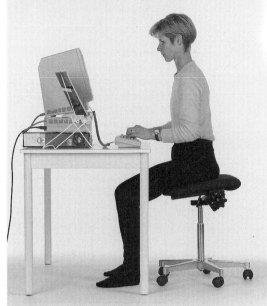

Fig. 91 The most frequent position for VDU operators: spot all the errors!

Fig. 92 Much improved ergonomics and body use: note use of copyholder.

least every hour for a few minutes; and every two to three hours lie in the balanced resting position for 10–20 minutes as part of a longer break (and make sure you don't work more than two of these 'shifts' a day). From time to time while at the computer let your eyes focus on distant objects to release the eye muscles responsible for focusing. Remember to let your eyes blink frequently and not stare at the screen.

If you suffer any symptoms of a repetitive strain injury, such as loss of power and movement, aching in the wrist, hands and fingers, burning sensations and so on, it is important to stop straight away. You have been overdoing it and – in all likelihood – misusing yourself as well. If you carry on you will be in serious trouble and you will need considerably more time off work or even be invalided out of your job. The good news is that if you can allow rest to heal the pathological changes which have taken place –

and that will be as long as it needs to be – you can learn to avoid the misuse which got you into trouble in the first place.

A typewriter poses its own difficulties. The keyboard is raked at a steep angle and the front of your desk may have a lip which limits how high you can sit and get your legs underneath. Bearing in mind the guiding principles suggested, make the best compromise you can. When playing a keyboard instrument, you have to balance the requirements of reaching the pedals with freedom of the arms.

Handwriting

We spend less time writing than a hundred years ago. None the less, school children still need to write, draw, use brushes, etc. for an appreciable part of the day. Students need fast and fluent penmanship and frequently get 'writer's cramp'. There are three aspects to consider: ergonomic factors; writing grips and, the most important of all, your general use.

Let's deal with some of the ergonomic factors first. You may want to look back over the section in this chapter on the working chair: a chair tilting you forwards from the hips will help bring you closer to your work. The other part of the equation is to bring your work closer to you. The writing surface needs to be roughly half your height (your arms can rest lightly on the desk to help avoid excessive tension in the arms and shoulders) and angled towards you: the writing surface should slope by approximately 15–20 degrees (*Fig. 93*). School desks used to slant, and we seem to have forgotten that a traditional design served – and may still serve – an important purpose.

You can improvise by putting blocks under the back of the desk to tilt the surface. Alternatively you can rest a large thin hardback or board on top of another book laid flat. Better still, purchase a writing slope or have one made (Appendix I).

What does writing require? Very simply, moving a small light object through small distances. In most offices or schools you can see the most extraordinary waste of energy in this task. Usually the whole body is slumped forwards, twisted and leaning to one side, the jaw is clamped, forehead furrowed, eyes staring, shoulders hunched, legs curled under the chair or round each other. Fingers are white, gripping the pen. A sizeable minority of adults have a callus near the end joint of the middle finger of their writing hand at some time.

Fig. 94 Paper placed level and slightly to the side helps avoid cramping of the arm and the need to twist the neck.

Fig. 93 Use of tilting chair and writing slope.

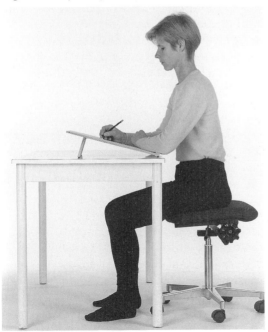

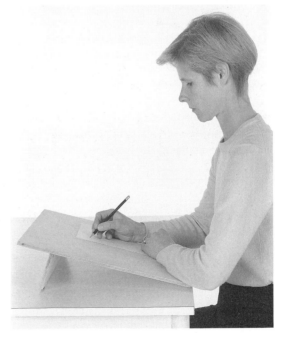

Body-use while writing

Ergonomic factors make an important difference, but they are not, of course, the whole answer. *The key factor is how you use yourself.*

Sit at a table or desk with paper and pencil. Notice if you slump and, if you are right-handed, if you tend to pull your head down to the left to look at the sheet of paper slanted to the left. Now the reason the paper is slanted is to give your writing arm space to move. If you straighten the paper in front of you to write you will probably find yourself leaning more over to the left to avoid the writing arm cramping. Ensure that you are sitting evenly over both sitting bones: the habit of leaning to one side is usually very strong.

Try placing the paper level and slightly to the right. Give directions and let your head tilt slightly forwards on top of your neck and then rotate your head a little to the right to see your work, thereby avoiding the twisting and pulling down to one side. Think of your neck and back tending back away from your work.

Using a writing slope (which has a small ledge to stop the paper sliding off), place your sheet of paper to the right (and any document to which you need to refer, to the left). Now begin to write (*Fig. 94*). Scan your body to see whether you can sense or observe undue effort and tension in any part. Notice if you are writing fluently and how much work is being done by your writing arm. If you have to write for any length of time use a pencil or fountain pen or their equivalents; ballpoint pens encourage tense grips.

Writing holds

I did not pay special attention to the way I held a pen until I became a mature student. Although I attended to the primary control while writing, I observed that my hold was tighter than it should be. What was wrong, I wondered?

I eventually came to the conclusion that there was something fundamentally wrong with my hold. Not that I was holding my pen in a particularly unusual grip – and there are some very strange ones! I held my pen between the pads of my thumb and first finger and against the lowest joint of my middle finger. This is how most children are taught how to hold a pen. However, if you take hold of the pen in this manner, it is almost impossible not to tighten the fingers – many bend the thumb to a right angle and the first finger is often bent back on itself or else hooked round the pen. Harmful pressure on the joint of the middle finger may lead to calluses. The wrist locks and there is a tendency to pull the elbow into the side and to clamp the upper arm into the shoulder. This kind of hold predisposes to the development of writer's cramp.

The alternative is to hold the pen between the pads of thumb, first and middle fingers, the other fingers loosely curled under and, with the heel of the hand, resting on the writing surface (*Fig. 95*). Note the link between this way of holding the pen and the hands on the chair-rail procedure. The fingers holding the pen should be lengthening and the shape of your hand in relation to your wrist is a 'beak'. Even though you may be familiar with this procedure, the new hold will feel very odd at first – as you would now expect of any radical change! Holding the pen in the familiar way since the age of five is bound to feel right and comfortable even though it may be very tense and produce cramp. We only have to *think* of writing and muscles respond as they always have done. How can this be changed?

The essential first step is to inhibit your immediate response to the idea of writing and to consider the means whereby freedom in the writing arm can be encouraged. The

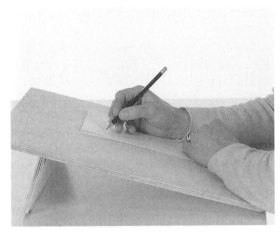

Fig. 95 Improved writing hold.

priority must be, of course, to release the neck and the arm will have the best possible chance of remaining free. With the writing hand resting on the desk in front of you as just described, give directions to the NHB relationship and then secondary directions to the shoulder, arm and fingers. Let the shoulder of the writing arm release and spread sideways, to let the extension continue out to the elbow. Let the hand ease out of the forearm and, as the fingers lengthen out of the hand, place the pen with your other hand between the pads of your thumb, index and middle fingers; continuing to let the fingers lengthen out of the hand, take hold of the pen gently but firmly.

Remind yourself that you do not intend to 'write', but to attend to the 'means-whereby'. It may be helpful to think of doodling or drawing simple shapes, instead. This is less likely to be associated with the particular tensions of writing and will help change your mind/body 'set'.

Putting it into practice

Now write your address and notice how your intention to write probably led you to hold the pen in your 'normal' manner. You will probably be in conflict between feeling out

of control (the new way) and wanting to remain in control (the habitual way). Be prepared to gradually give up your old control and you will eventually find a new one!

Beware of your thumb flexing unduly (it will tighten and the wrist will lock): there should be some movement of the thumb, but it should be balanced by movements of the index and middle fingers to control the pen. Let your whole arm move freely across the paper, elbow leading, avoiding excessive movement of the wrist joint. If you need to increase the pressure of your writing, much less effort will be made if you direct your fingers down into the paper as you think of your spine lengthening upwards.

Fig. 96 Erasmus by Quentin Metsys, 1517 (by permission of H.M. The Queen). Note the expanded posture, the head tilted forward on top of the neck, the use of a sloped writing surface and the correct hold. Erasmus wrote In Praise of Folly *in a few days!* (Photo: The Royal Collection)

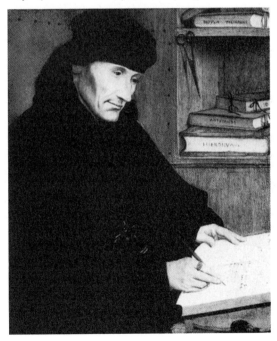

Here is another demonstration of how your thinking directly conditions your muscular responses. Suppose that at work you need to get a handwritten note dashed off. You may forget everything about the Alexander Technique on that occasion! In time, though, you can endeavour to make steady improvement. When you have a spare moment, practice the procedure suggested above. The freer hold will begin to carry over more and more into your writing. A cramped writing style will change to a larger, more fluent style. This new hold is invaluable for anyone using shorthand.

My conjecture is that this manner of holding a pen used to be routinely taught up to the end of the last century. Martineau (1826–69) painted 'Kit's Writing Lesson' in which a young child is shown struggling to master this craft. Apart from the strain shown on his unwilling face, what is interesting is that the hold shown is exactly as I have described it. No doubt he would have had his knuckles rapped had he held his pen incorrectly! There are also striking portraits of Erasmus by Holbein and Metsys which illustrate clearly many of the points made.

Brushing your teeth

There are, of course, many other situations where gripping an implement tightly is quite unnecessary. A good example is brushing your teeth. Part of most people's early morning ritual – usually performed with minimal awareness – why not give it some attention? (It will give you clues as to how you hold practically anything!) You will probably

Fig. 97 Moving your head against the brush, everything tightening!

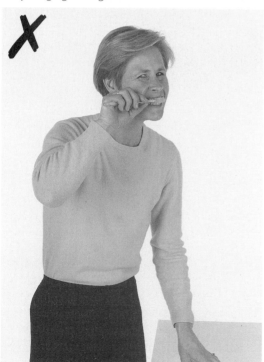

Fig. 98 Brushing your teeth with free arm and neck.

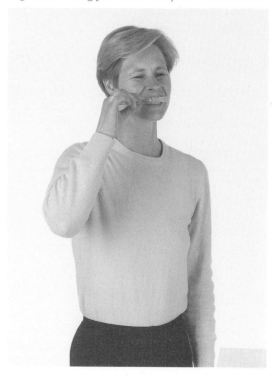

Fig. 99

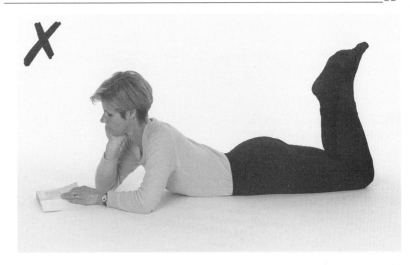

Fig. 100

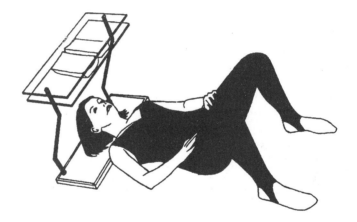

notice that you clench the handle in the palm of your hand, fingers tightened around the toothbrush, producing an inordinate amount of tension in your whole arm and shoulder (*Fig. 97*). You may even be using your head to move your teeth against the brush!

To change this you need to begin by paying attention to the primary control. Before picking up the toothbrush, renew your directions and then hold it lightly with the ends of the fingers, letting your shoulder release sideways, the extension continuing out to your elbow. This will provide all the pressure you need and protect your gums

from excessive abrasion (*Fig. 98*).

Reading

The point is to have your reading material sufficiently high and close to you so that you can tilt your head forwards on the neck without collapsing forwards. Sitting in an armchair you can rest your book on substantial cushions. At a desk, use a copyholder. Lying down, try to avoid propping your head up on your arms (*Fig. 99*). There are alternatives, but unfortunately you have to lift the book up to turn the pages! (*Fig. 100*)

Driving

Do you suffer from pain across the base of the neck and shoulders or from headaches when driving long distances or when you are in a hurry to get somewhere? If so, your body-use and your driving position are suspect.

Seat adjustment

At one end of the range, taller people have trouble because there is not sufficient head clearance in many cars. At the other end, shorter people strain to peer over the steering wheel. Comfort in driving over long periods ought to be a major part of any decision to purchase a particular model of car. For a short person, the situation is easily remedied by a wedge-shaped cushion. For a tall person who scrunches down, the solution (more expensive, usually!) is to change your car.

The most common errors in seat adjustment are as follows. The anxious driver tends to grip the wheel too fiercely – as if it were about to be wrestled from their grip – and to sit, cramped, too close to the controls (*Fig. 101*). The laid-back driver, in reclining too much, pulls forward and down to reach the controls (*Fig. 102*). Both tend to suffer undue fatigue and discomfort and – most seriously – lapses of attention.

The seat should be close enough to the controls so that you can reach them without having to lean forwards away from the back of the seat to change into first gear or to operate a hand-brake. You can monitor this by feeling the upper part of your back losing contact with the seat back (*Fig. 103*).

On the other hand, you should not be so close that you get 'accelerator foot' on the motorway – when the ankle is so flexed that discomfort and undue tension set in. Sit far enough away from the foot pedals so that the angles made at hips, knees and ankles

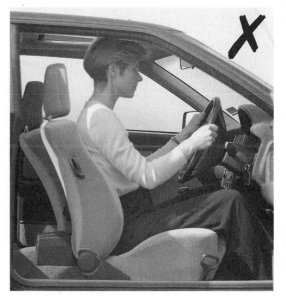

Fig. 101 Cramped driving position.

are all open angles – greater than 90 degrees. The seat should recline slightly to maintain this open angle between torso and thigh. The slightest lumbar curve should be preserved; a lumbar roll or strongly curved back support – unless the seat back is very concave – will probably cause the lumbar spine to arch excessively. A small cushion can be useful in supporting the pelvis and lower/middle back.

Improved use when driving

Place your sitting bones as far back in the seat as possible, weight evenly over both of them and let as much of your back as possible stay back against the seat. Sitting in a car for any length of time is a good opportunity to give the directions: remember to keep releasing the neck to let the head go forwards and upwards and the back to lengthen and widen and flatten out against the seat back. Direct your knees forward and slightly apart from each other out over the feet, so that your leg joints are all hinging in the same plane on each side. When you

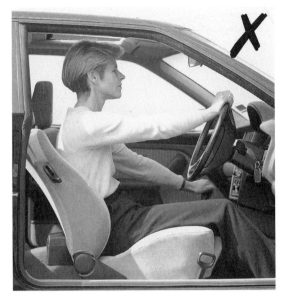

Fig. 102 *Too laid back!*

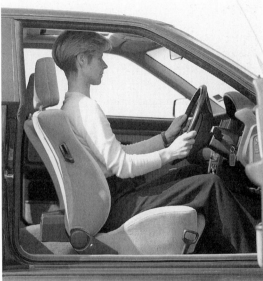

Fig. 103 *Improved driving position.*

move your legs or arms, remember to think of them moving away from your torso.

You will need to lean forward away from the back of the seat in certain circumstances. You come to a road junction. This is often a time of anxiety: the neck stiffens, but you need to turn your head quickly from side to side. Think your neck free and lean forwards from your hips, letting the head curve forwards and up. Your eye level will drop slightly below horizontal. Renew letting go of the neck and allow the head to turn around a forward tilting axis to check the road, thereby avoiding the pulling back of the head into the shoulders. Awareness of traffic conditions must of course be maintained!

Another situation is reversing your car in order to park. There are limits as to how far the head will turn, and – rather than wrench the head round – remove your safety belt and shift your whole body a little way round in the direction you need to look so that you will be able to turn your head easily without strain.

Now for the steering wheel. It used to be standard practice for learners to be instructed to hold the wheel at the ten-to-two or quarter-to-three position. This actually speeds the onset of fatigue and increases arm, neck and shoulder tension, thereby slowing your reactions. It is preferable to hold the wheel in a looser way by the base of the first three fingers – other fingers wrapped loosely round the wheel – at a quarter-to-four or twenty-to-five position. Note the similarity to the heels of the hands resting on the chair-rail procedure and give directions accordingly. This should help you be more alert and able to react faster in an emergency. When parking or turning a sharp corner, move the hands up the wheel and use all the fingers of the hand as appropriate to turn the wheel (don't wrestle with it!).

Cycling

Dropped handlebars – even with levers on the handlebars – should be avoided: to monitor traffic, your head is inevitably going to jam back on your neck into your shoulders. In the final analysis, it comes down to your priorities. The legs certainly work more powerfully in this racing position, but at great cost to the neck and back. Sacrificing some loss of power by using straighter handlebars will mean you will be able to cycle well into the 21st century with ease and comfort – and have a safer view of the traffic!

Frame size and shape are important considerations. Cyclists commonly have bikes too small for them so that they are more likely to hunch over the handlebars. The design of mountain bikes seems to encourage this. Women's bicycles are often built with a long frame base so that it is impossible to avoid leaning a long way forward.

The bike doesn't need to be the 'sit up and beg' type: a slight lean forwards from the hips is quite acceptable. Remember to let the head nod forwards slightly on top of the neck to allow the back to lengthen. Let the shoulders release and spread sideways to allow the elbows to curve sideways so that the arms make a shallow, expanding circle, the back staying back away from the handlebars.

There are often misconceptions about the best height of the saddle. The criterion to be used should not in general be: can I get my feet on the ground, sitting on the saddle?

The legs will be too cramped and tire very easily, and you will be more tempted to bend the back to try to get more power into the legs. Instead, with one pedal at the bottom of its travel – and the ball of the foot on the pedal – the saddle should be high enough to allow the leg *almost* to straighten, but not to lock the knee.

When you cycle, allow your legs to move *from* the hips without tilting them from side to side. This tends to happen when the saddle is too high and the lower back then twists. The torso should remain quite still.

The final thing to consider is your knees. The knees are commonly pulled in towards each other in cycling, especially in women; and the feet are often splayed outwards. The thighs tend to jam into the hips. Knee and ankle joints will be stressed because they are working at the edge of the range of their movement, and the downwards thrust of the leg will be less efficient. Of course, when you direct your knees out over your feet, your initial *feeling* will probably be that your knees are too wide apart!

When you cycle up a steep gradient and stand on the pedals, you do not need to shorten your spine as you pull up on the handlebars: keep the opposition going between the thrust of the legs downwards and the lengthening of the spine upwards and leave your shoulders free.

CHAPTER 9

Are you a top-heavy mover?

Place a small object on the floor just in front of you at an angle to a mirror and then pick it up slowly. Try to see how you bend and compare that with what you can register kinaesthetically. You will probably notice that your legs tend to stiffen and toes clench as you bend over and hunch your back. Pause for a moment as you pick up the object and notice also how tense the neck

Fig. 104 Top-heavy, twisted bending.

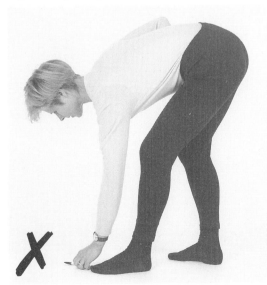

has become; even if you bent your knees a little, the heels may have come off the floor. If you put one leg forwards and used the arm on the same side of the body to pick up the object, the back twists as well as collapsing and is therefore especially vulnerable. This is one example of 'top-heavy' movement (*Figs. 104 and 105*).

You may be thinking, 'Surely it doesn't really matter if I lift a *light* object in a top-heavy way?' If you think carefully about it, though, you are conditioning yourself to the idea of bending in a malcoordinated way. When you come to lift a more substantial load, even if you remember the standard instruction – bend your knees! – muscles will respond according to the usual habit of bending (*Fig. 106*).

This kind of misuse, continually repeated, leads to cumulative strain and can cause disabling back problems. What seems to be a trivial bending movement can be 'the straw that breaks the camel's back'. The connection between what we do and its consequences may appear tenuous. (It can take 24 hours or so before damage to the intervertebral disc is registered. The disc has no direct nerve supply and it takes time for the diffusion of certain chemicals released by

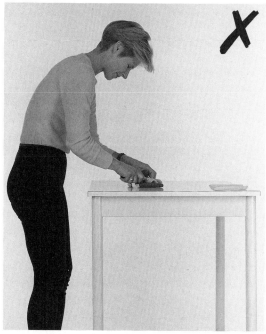

Fig. 105 Housework can produce much pulling down.

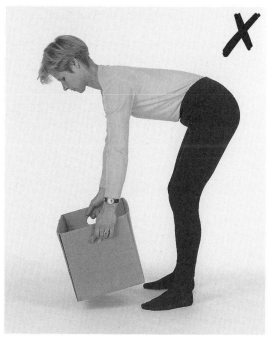

Fig. 106 How to damage your back in one careless movement!

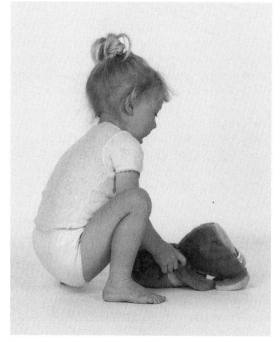

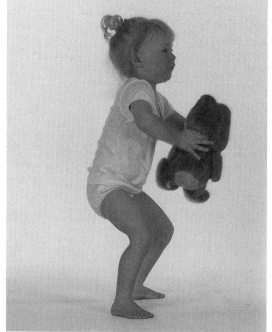

Figs. 107 and 108 The toddler shows a supple and easy use of the legs.

damage to act on nearby nerve fibres.)

Contrast this kind of bending and lifting with that of a toddler. Hips, knees and ankles bend freely, the legs work powerfully and the proper relationship between head, neck and back is undisturbed. What's more, the youngster can stay in a deep squat for long periods of time with ease (*Figs. 107 and 108*).

Discovering your hip joints

The hip joints are – after the atlanto-occipital joint – the most important joints to locate and to use properly. When bending, we should recover our ability to hinge at the hips, knees and ankles just like the child! The hip joints are in fact *lower* than we may realize. Our image of where we should bend is often somewhere between the pelvis and waist and this is where we tend to bend – by collapsing the back in this region.

While standing, raise and lower one knee a little. Feel where the hip joint is at the front of your leg by having a good dig around at the top of the thigh just beneath the bony pelvis; at the back of the thigh, the hip joint can be felt just in front of the sitting bone. This practical knowledge will help you understand where bending should begin.

There are two procedures for rehearsing the kind of bending which should take place in many of our daily activities: the 'monkey' and the 'lunge'. *Again your teacher will introduce you to these procedures so that you understand them properly*. These 'positions of mechanical advantage' – as Alexander originally called them – can be modified in all sorts of ways depending on the particular task to be carried out. We will focus on the 'monkey' first.

Monkey

This way of bending was soon abbreviated to 'monkey' by Alexander's students for obvious reasons as you will see! The monkey is usually demonstrated with feet about a hips-to-shoulders width apart. Depending on its practical application, the feet could also be placed together or considerably wider apart. The monkey should be used, for instance, when washing up, or washing the hands or face, or when lifting relatively stable objects such as shopping bags or boxes, or in sports like skiing, skating, tennis, horse-riding and the martial arts.

The monkey is normally rehearsed in two stages at the beginning because to go directly from standing to bending forward normally produces a considerable amount of misuse – pulling forwards and down (*Fig. 109*). The first stage, therefore, is to let the legs bend as you lengthen upwards along the spine. And the forward inclination is achieved by letting the head lead the torso forward and up in a curved movement out of the hips while you let the knees bend a little more (*Figs. 110–112*).

Let's examine the monkey in detail. You will probably begin from a standing position with feet close together. Give directions to the primary control and, while lengthening, lift one knee a little to place the foot about a hips-to-shoulders width apart from the other one. Check that the feet are pointing slightly outwards in line with the forward-and-apart direction the knees will release when bending.

1) Renew the directions: in the context of growing up along the spine, establish the opposition between the head going forward and up and the neck and back going back and up. This will tend to carry the hips slightly backwards. Let the knees release very slightly forwards. You are thereby 'priming' the proper oppositional forces within the body which can then inform the movement (*Fig. 110*).

Fig. 109 Pulling forwards and down.

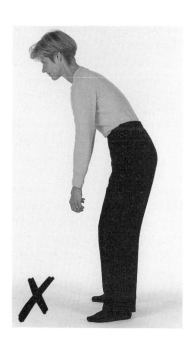

Figs. 110–112 Going into monkey.

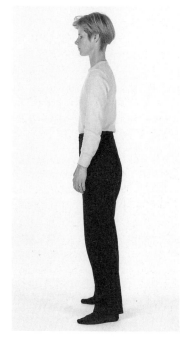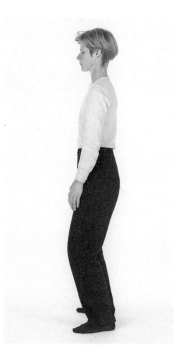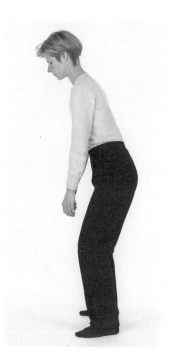

2) As you continue lengthening upwards, let the back tend back as you allow your knees to bend forwards and slightly apart from each other (*Fig. 111*). At first only bend your knees a little; later on you will be able to bend lower and lower without pulling down (*Figs. 113 and 114*).

Common errors include pulling the knees together with the hips thrusting forwards. If you check in a mirror, you will see a sway-back (*Fig. 115*). Another 'different kind of badly' is to pull forwards and down, sticking out and tightening the buttocks, and hollowing the lower back (*Fig. 116*).

The key to the monkey is – while lengthening along the spine – to let the back widen – letting the hips stay back in relation to the knees going forward as the legs fold underneath you. Body weight should stay centred over the centre of the feet.

3) The final stage of the monkey is to lean forwards from the hips. Let the head lead in a curving forwards and up trajectory (from the top of the neck), neck and back following, letting the knees – and ankles and hips – bend slightly as the torso inclines forwards from the hips (*Fig. 112*). If you don't let your leg joints release properly, the weight will shift forwards onto the front of your feet, your toes will clench, your buttocks raise and your lower back hollow. Your eye level should drop so that you look at the floor some feet in front of you. Your arms should hang freely. With your lower back releasing and expanding, breathing should be freer.

Monkey against a wall

To help you get a better idea of the importance of the whole of the back staying back in this movement, use the help of a wall. This will, of course, exaggerate the 'back back' aspect of the monkey, but it may make it

Fig. 113

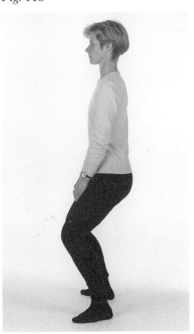

Fig. 114

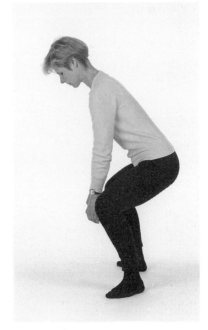

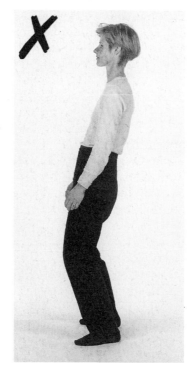
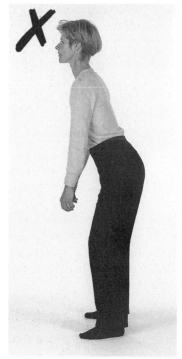

Fig. 115 Showing 'swayback'.
Fig. 116 Far right

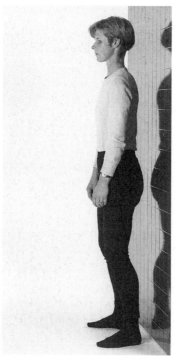
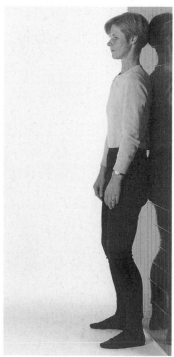

Figs. 117–120 right Monkey against a wall sequence.

easier for you to make this connection in the free-standing situation.

1) Stand about 2 inches away from a smooth wall or door (or less, if there is a skirting board), feet a hips-to-shoulders width apart. Give directions to the NHB relationship (*Fig. 117*).

2) While directing the head forwards and up, lean back releasing the hips and ankles so that you make contact with the surface behind you at approximately the same time with buttocks and shoulder blades (*Fig. 118*). (The weight will now be further back on the heels than in the free-standing situation.)

3) Give directions to the primary control and let the knees bend forwards and slightly apart from each other, letting the back flatten closer to the surface behind you, leaning *lightly* against it (*Fig. 119*).

If you pull forward and down, you will feel the upper back losing contact with the surface. *This is how most people bend their knees – pushing them down into their feet – rather than letting the leg joints hinge freely as the spine lengthens upwards.* So pay attention to the upper back staying back – while letting the head tend *forward* and up – and also let the lower back ease more and more into contact with the wall as the knees bend, allowing the pelvis to tilt back. (Note the similarity to the lying down releasing position.)

4) To lean forwards from the hips, remember to stop and give directions to the neck, head and back. Then let the head lead in a curved forwards and up direction as you let the knees release a small amount forwards, hips and ankles bending. The buttocks stay lightly in contact with the door or wall (*Fig. 120*). The weight should now again be over

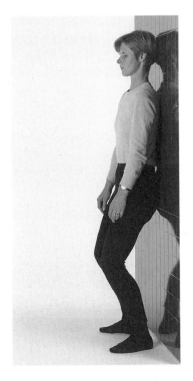

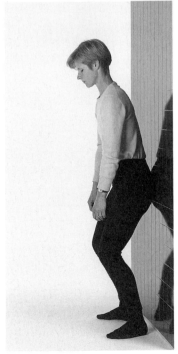

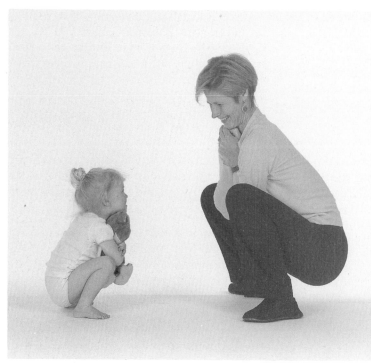

Fig. 121 The adult can relearn to squat as easily as the young child!

Figs. 122–124 right Going into a squat.

the feet arches (if it is not, adjust the feet in relation to the wall next time).

5) To return to a standing position, while directing the head forwards and up, allow the neck and back to move back and up so that you are once more in contact with the wall.

6) Then let the head ease forwards and up from between the shoulders, torso following and sliding up against the wall, legs straightening last (don't forget to let the knees remain unlocked when you come to standing).

7) Letting the head lead forward and up, let your weight shift forwards off the heels to a balanced position over the whole of the feet; you are now back where you started.

Squatting

Toddlers easily squat. This is how people in some cultures usually sit – squatting on their haunches. (Degenerative osteoarthritic changes of the hips in these cultures is largely unknown.) A large degree of flexibility in the hips, knees and ankles is required for this, much of which is lost as we get older – but not irrevocably so. Heels staying down provide more thrust to the upward movement in lifting so that the big thigh muscles can do most of the work. The lengthening back muscles will protect the back from damage (*Fig. 121*).

Going into a squat is basically a series of lower and lower monkeys. One way is to go into the first stage of the monkey, lengthening upwards to bend the knees as far as you can without pulling down. You will be able to bend to a certain level where the ankles will flex no further (*Fig. 122*). At this point you could let the heels come off the floor but your balance would be precarious and your lower back would tend to arch.

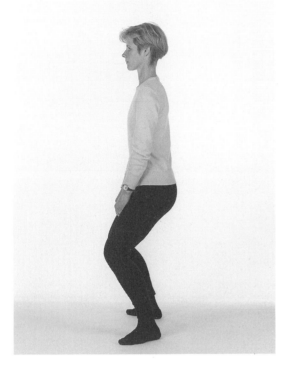

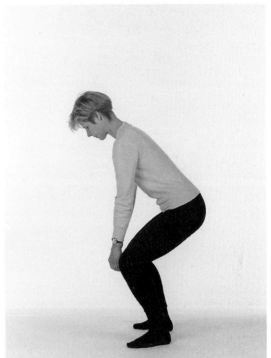

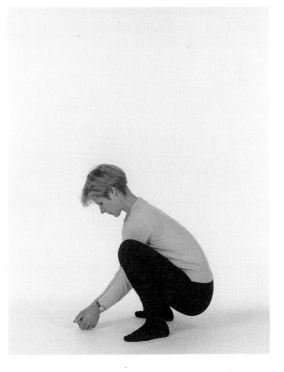

Instead, let the head curve forwards and up to lean forwards from the hips and let the knees bend a little further. By letting the leg joints release and by leaning slightly further forwards each time from the hips (letting the weight remain over the centre of the feet, you will gradually be able to get lower and lower (*Fig. 123*). Do not force this movement – be patient! It may take a long time to get right down to a deep squat and to be able to stay there for some time in reasonable comfort without tightening the ankles (*Fig. 124*).

The point of the Alexander Technique is to be free and lengthening in any position, not whether the 'shape' looks ideally correct. On occasion movements need to be made which are less mechanically advisable. Aim to do your best in the circumstances you find yourself.

In everyday movement, you would go straight into the second stage of the monkey and progressively lean slightly further

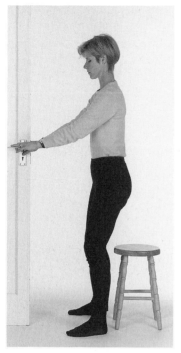

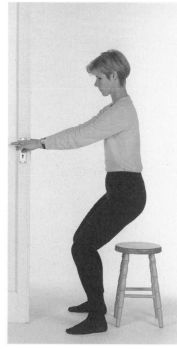

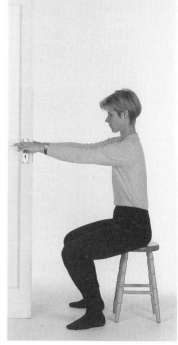

Fig. 125   *Fig. 126*   *Fig. 127*

forwards as you let the legs fold underneath you.

The flexibility of the lower limbs in squatting is far more important to maintain or recover than touching your toes. It will help protect your back from damage when lifting or gardening and in your old age you will still be able to cut your toe nails!

Squatting procedure using door handles
To help extend the range of leg flexion you can utilize a half-open door, holding the handles to help you balance as you lean back and upwards to let the knees bend. This movement takes you further back than it is possible to do so when free standing, but it is valuable for giving you more experience of letting your back stay in relation to head and knees.

1) With the door open, stand a hips-to-shoulders width apart facing the edge of the door, and close enough to be able to gently grasp the handles with arms straight (but without locking the elbows). A chair should be placed just behind you so that it touches the back of the legs. Lengthening upwards and letting the back stay back, move one arm at a time to take hold of the door handles (*Fig. 125*).

2) As you direct the head forwards and up, think the neck and back back, letting the hips release backwards as you bend the knees forwards and apart from each other out over the feet, maintaining length in the spine. You should now find yourself sitting in an upright position (*Figs. 126 and 127*).

Monitor what happened: if your real concern was to sit down in the chair and you forget about the primary control, you will probably arrive in the chair leaning forwards, hips further back than the

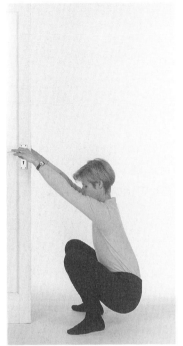

Fig. 128

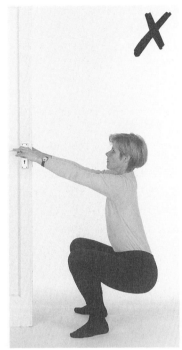

Fig. 129

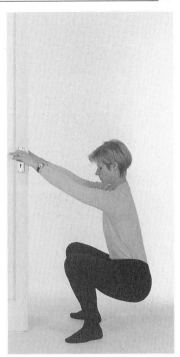

Fig. 130

shoulders and the back hollowed! A delicate balance between all the opposing forces is required for this movement to work well.

3) To return to standing, more work needs to be done by the legs than in a free-standing position. As you direct your head forwards and up, lean back and up out of the hips away from the door. Drive your feet down into the floor, sending the knees forwards and apart. Release your shoulders to spread sideways; arms should remain lengthened and not contract to pull you up. Continue renewing the directions and you will find yourself suddenly lifting off the chair to reach a standing position once more.

4) The next stage is to employ a lower chair or stool. Finally you will be able to go down onto your haunches into a deep squat (*Fig. 128*). To return to standing, as before, avoid pulling yourself up by tightening (*Fig. 129*).

Follow the instructions in (3) again (*Fig. 130*).

The lunge

This bending position has the feet placed approximately a hips-width apart and one in front of the other, providing a powerful base for shifting body weight forwards or backwards. You will need a teacher to guide you properly through the procedure. The lunge is useful for any pulling or pushing movements. Applications include pushing and pulling a trolley; sweeping; vacuuming; ironing; opening and closing a door; and in various sports such as tennis, fencing and the martial arts. With the feet closer together, knees slightly bent, you have a stance more useful than a wide monkey when you are standing at a work surface (*Fig. 131*).

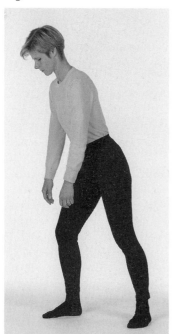

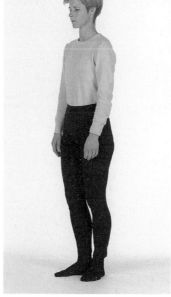

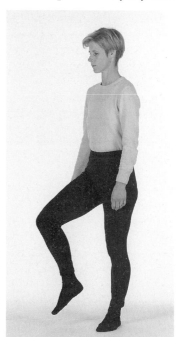

Fig. 131

Fig. 132

Fig. 133

Fig. 134

Fig. 135

Fig. 136

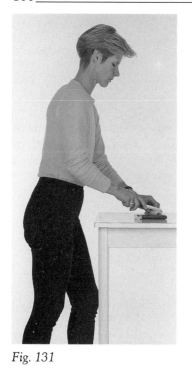

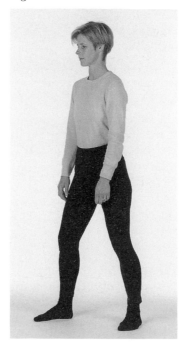

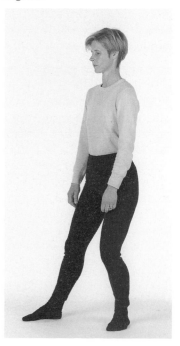

Like the monkey, the lunge is shown by the teacher in a number of stages to clarify the elements of the movement. Used in everyday activities, the distinction between one movement and the next is often blurred or parts of the lunge as described here are omitted altogether (*Figs. 132–39*).

1) Being in a standing position, feet close together. Lengthening upwards, transfer the weight to one leg (let the knee bend slightly), turn the head, neck and torso on the hips about 30 degrees, placing the heel of the foot of the 'empty' leg against the instep of the leg you are standing on. You should now be facing – hips square on – the direction you want to lunge towards, front foot also pointing in that direction, back foot at about a 30 degree angle (*Fig. 140*).

2) Renew the directions, lifting the knee of the 'empty' leg up away from the lower back and a little to the side (to lunge to a forward position, with the feet a hips-width apart) (*Fig. 141*).

3) To lunge, let the head lead the torso in a curving forwards and up direction and *then* let the foot drop softly down about a foot or two in advance of the other, letting the front knee bend; most of your weight is then transferred to the front leg. Be prepared to lose your balance rather than stiffen in the attempt to maintain it. Keep lengthening along your spine! Check that the front foot reaches the floor at the equivalent of about a hips-width apart (although forward, of course, from the back leg). Let the joints in the front leg release sufficiently so that the toes do not clench and so that the weight is distributed equally over the sole of that foot (*Fig. 142*).

4) To draw backwards, the head needs to be

Fig. 137

Fig. 138

Fig. 139

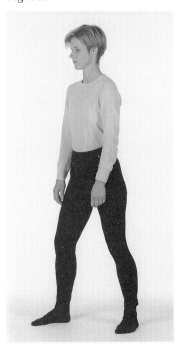

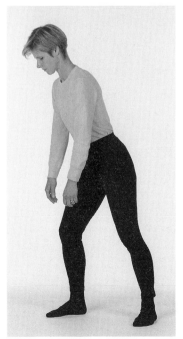

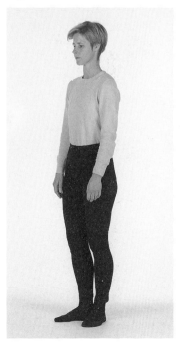

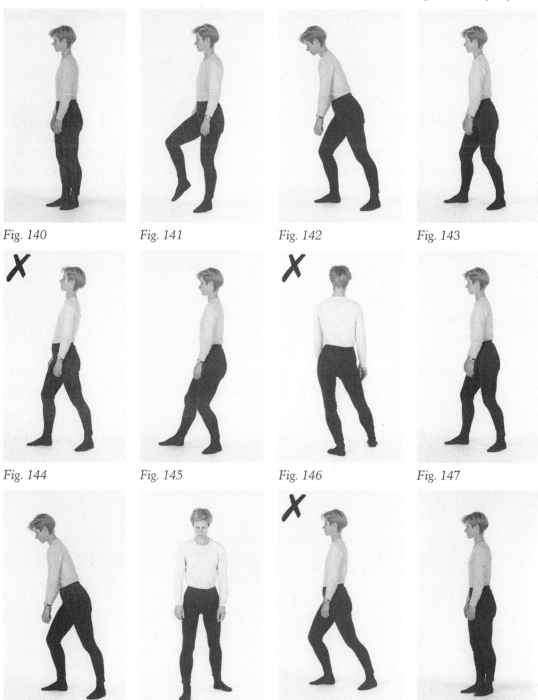

Fig. 140

Fig. 141

Fig. 142

Fig. 143

Fig. 144

Fig. 145

Fig. 146

Fig. 147

Fig. 148

Fig. 149

Fig. 150

Fig. 151

directed forwards and up; let the neck and back draw back and up as the front leg almost straightens (the knee remains 'soft'). You will now have slightly more of your weight on the back leg – knee slightly bent (*Fig. 143*). Avoid pulling your head back which arches the back and loses the power of the movement (*Fig. 144*).

5) To go 'down' (that is, to bend the back leg), direct your head to go forwards and up to lengthen your spine and let your neck and back draw back and up to let the back knee bend out over the foot (*Fig. 145*). A common error is to sway back and push the hip sideways so that the lower back twists (*Fig. 146*). If the knee cannot bend much when you first try this, so be it. It is more important for the hips to remain square throughout the sequence and the back not to twist.

6) The next phase of the movement is to lengthen upwards to 'straighten' the back leg – but leaving a slight bend in the knee – by letting the head lead in a forwards and up movement (*Fig. 147*). Avoid pulling the head back and raising the chest.

7) To shift the weight forward, the sequence of movement is to let the head curve forwards and up away from the back heel, which drives down into the floor – straightening the leg – and the front knee bends passively out over the foot (*Figs. 148 and 149*). In T'ai Chi terminology, the back leg is active, helping to thrust you forwards and the front leg passively 'fills up' as the knee bends. This is a powerful movement. If, however, the front knee is active – pushing you forward – the lower back will hollow and you lose most of the power of your shifting body weight, as well as putting more strain on your back (*Fig. 150*). If the knee turns inwards, you will twist the back. (It is possible, of course, to turn the whole torso

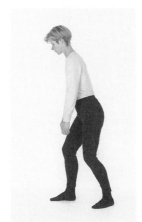
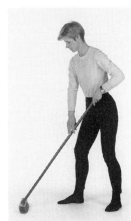

Fig. 152   Fig. 153

on the hips a *small* distance without twisting the back.)

8) To return to where you began, remind yourself to leave the neck alone. Let the head go forwards and up as you thrust backwards off the front leg, so that as the front leg 'empties', the back leg 'fills' and the front knee can then be lifted to bring the feet close together again (*Fig. 151*).

When you have mastered the various stages of this movement, it will be relatively easy to merge the movements into each other, shifting the weight forwards and backwards as required. Often you won't need to lean so far forwards from the hips if at all: you can let the back knee bend as well as the front knee (*Fig. 152*). In this way you can see the application of the lunge to activities such as vacuuming or sweeping. The power of the body weight shifting forwards or drawing back should produce most of the movement of the vacuum cleaner or brush; arms and shoulders have a secondary, guiding role. Remember that your legs give you a strong flexible base. Adjust the feet as needed in order to point the front foot in the direction you are going, hips remaining square on (*Fig. 153*).

Getting into and out of chairs

Getting into and out of a chair usually involves a considerable amount of misuse. Refining the quality of this oft-repeated movement through inhibition and direction is a surprisingly big challenge. (Much time is spent in most teacher-training courses of the Alexander Technique on 'chair-work'.)

Getting out of a chair

1) Let's begin sitting on the chair. Sitting at ease, you would normally use the back of the chair – if adequate – for support. However, to get out of a chair, the further back you sit and the lower the chair and the further forward your feet are, the more you are likely to pull forwards and down. To get yourself to the front of the chair, stop and give directions and bring the arms back one by one to the arm rests or to take hold of the sides of the back of the chair. Letting the head lead forwards and up, use the arms and the feet driving down to help lift yourself to the edge of the chair (*Fig. 154*). (This approach is particularly useful to help get out of a very low chair.)

2) Bring your arms forwards to place your hands – apart – on your lap (hands together or resting on knees will tend to pull you down). Place the feet so that one is under the chair (that heel will be off the floor), the other drawn close to the chair with the heel on or very close to the floor, knees apart (*Fig. 155*).

3) To lean forwards from the hips, let the neck release to let the head curve forwards and up to lengthen the spine and let the directions inform the movement; the eyes will be looking down a few feet in front of you. Avoid using momentum – throwing the chest out, the chin up and hollowing the

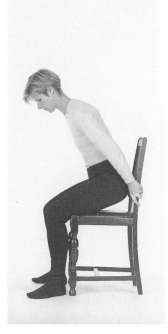

Getting out of a chair.

Fig. 154

lower back – to make this movement (*Fig.156*).

As you lean forward in the appropriate way, you will reach a position where, as Alexander described it – should the chair be removed – you would be performing a 'frog dance'!; or, continuing to lean forwards from the hips, you could reach forwards and pick something up off the floor (*Figs. 157 and 158*). *In other words, you have not committed yourself to the end of getting out of the chair, the idea of which is associated in the mind with certain muscular contractions. Instead, the process by which you will in time be able to arise from the chair with less and less effort, is the important thing.*

4) Direct the neck to release again to let the head lead forward and up and, as the weight moves over the feet, continue sending the knees forwards and apart and let the legs straighten, head leading, body following.

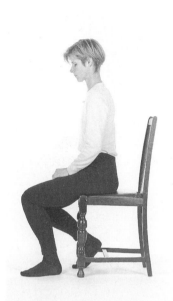

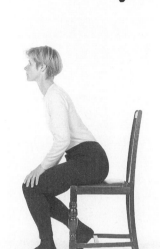

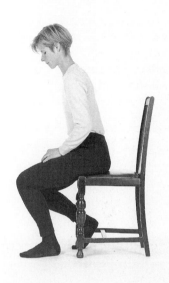

Fig. 155

Fig. 158

Fig. 156 How not to get out of a
chair – using excessive tension.
Fig. 159

Fig. 157

Fig. 160

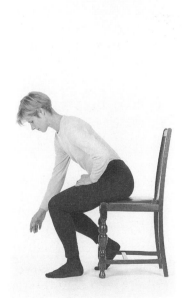

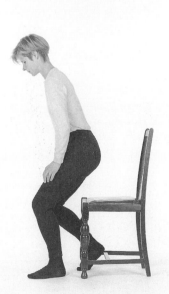

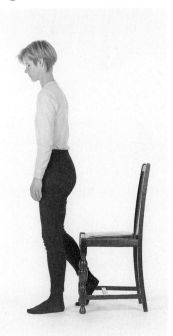

How to sit down.

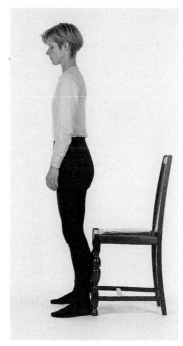

Fig. 161

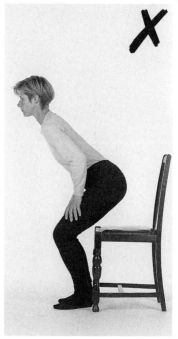

Fig. 162 *The wrong way.*

Inhibit any tendency to pull the knees in to engage the legs. As you come to a standing position, remember to renew your directions (*Figs. 159 and 160*). (At any moment you can switch off or you have an opportunity to be present!).

Sitting down
To sit down without the usual pulling down. it is necessary – as always – to bear in mind the 'means whereby'; let the chair interrupt your descent, rather than reaching for the chair with the buttocks. Sitting down is a series of lower and lower monkeys.

1) Stand with the feet about a hips-to-shoulders-width apart, backs of the legs close to the seat of the chair. Or with the feet apart as before and with one slightly behind the other, more weight on the front leg, back heel off the floor to get the foot further underneath the chair. Order the neck to

relax, the head to go forwards and up, and the back to lengthen and widen so that the lower back tends to swell out (*Fig. 161*).

2) Now there are two ways of getting the hips back, necessary for the sitting bones to be over the chair: you can merely push the hips back – this will be accompanied by a tendency to pull forwards and down – the movement we make habitually (*Fig. 162*); alternatively, *the hips can move back as a consequence of the back widening* (Fig. 163).

3) As the legs fold underneath you – knees forwards and apart – continue directing the head forward and upward to maintain the lengthening of the spine and the widening of the back. You will then find yourself sitting in the chair, leaning slightly forwards (*Fig. 164*).

4) To sit upright, pause: renew the directions and let yourself hinge backwards from

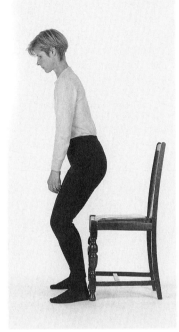

Fig. 163

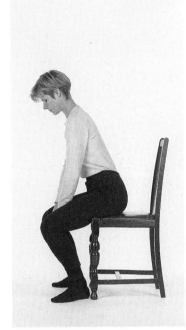

Fig. 164

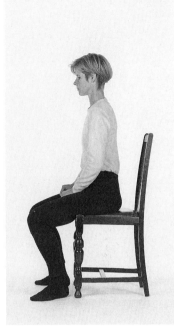

Fig. 165

Fig. 166 Top heavy bending.

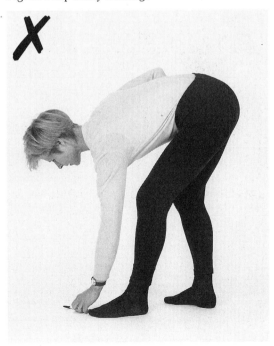

the hips, head going forwards and up as the neck and back ease back and upward (*Fig. 165*). (Note that 'forward and up' keeps changing in orientation as the angle of the body alters.)

So the act of sitting is the same as arising out of a chair – but in reverse. The only film record of F.M. Alexander at work (made in the late 1940s, close to his 80th birthday) – which has recently been transcribed onto video – can be seen in reverse. It is impossible to tell whether he is taking his pupils into or out of the chair.

Lifting and carrying

Some basic guidelines first. Carry the load close to your centre of gravity. Let your legs provide an adjustable, powerful base so that the arms and shoulders and lower back take little strain. Lengthen as you lift, leaving the

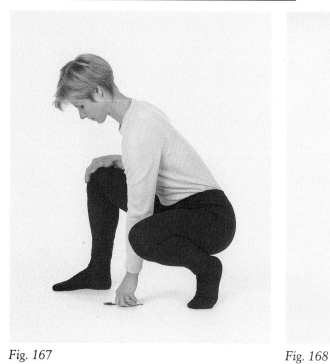

Fig. 167

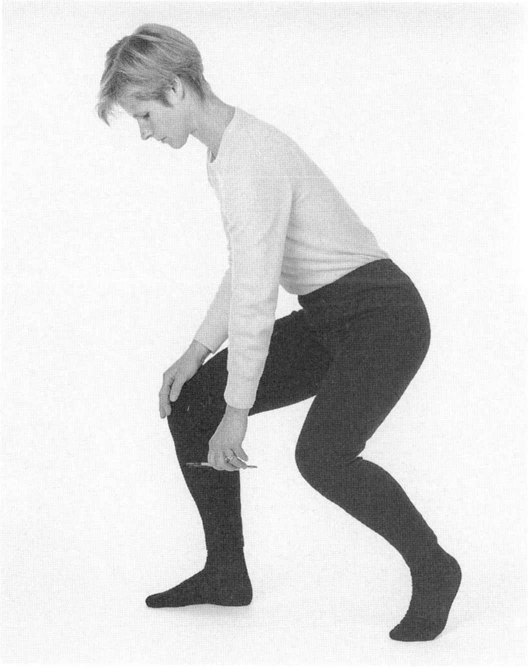

Fig. 168

Fig. 169

Fig. 170

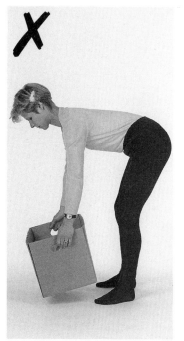

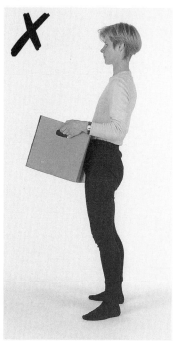

Fig. 169–170 Strained lifting technique

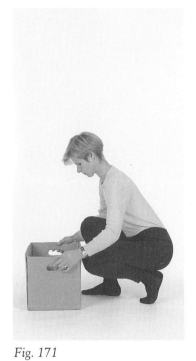

Fig. 171

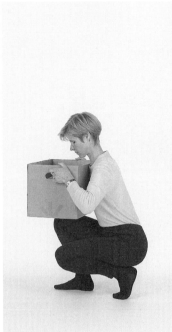

Fig. 172

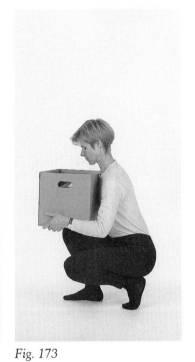

Fig. 173

Fig. 174

Figs. 171–174 Economical lifting technique.

Fig. 175

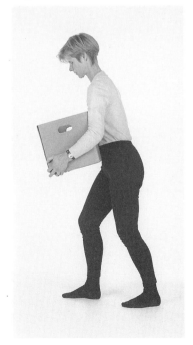

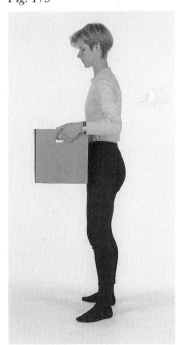

Right: Balanced carrying.

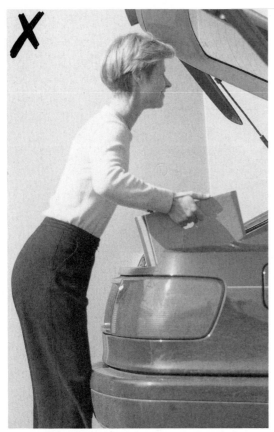

Fig. 176 *How to let shopping break your back!*

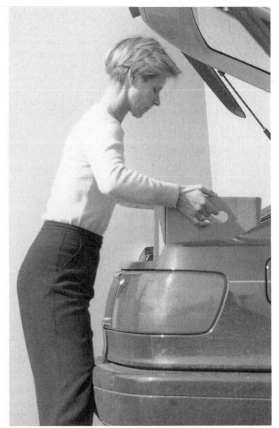

Fig. 177 *Doing the best of a difficult job.*

neck free – rather than tightening and contracting – whether the object is light or heavy.

You will recall mention of the need to prevent 'top-heavy' bending at the beginning of the chapter (*Fig. 166*). When bending to the floor, until you can manage a full squat, use a half squat, back heel lifting off the floor (*Figs. 167 and 168*). Also contrast the strain in lifting a heavy box (*Figs. 169 and 170*) with a more intelligent coordinated approach (*Figs. 171–174*). When you carry a load, beware of swaying back. Let the knees remain 'soft' when standing or walking as you let your back lengthen and widen (*Fig. 175*).

Sometimes difficult compromises have to be made. Getting shopping into and out of a car boot is potentially very hazardous for the back. It may be possible to rest your knee on the car bumper to reduce the amount of leaning forward. When that isn't possible, if you stiffen your legs, you are going to be in trouble (*Fig. 176*). Alternatively, place your legs wider apart to bend your knees and let the primary control and thighs do the work (*Fig. 177*).

Carrying shopping: if you can't use a trolley, distribute the load between two bags rather than carrying one heavy bag, which will pull you down on one side. Before you hurry off, pause for a moment. Oppose the downward pull by thinking up along your spine, leaving your neck free. Let the shoulders widen and the arms hang to distribute the weight into the back rather than being pulled down.

Carrying a rucksack: the shoulder straps will tend to pull you back and down, hollowing your back. Make sure you use the strap usually provided to go round your waist and that the shoulder straps are properly adjusted. As you walk, lean very slightly forwards from your hips, letting your lower back swell out backwards as you lengthen along the spine.

Pregnancy and childbirth

This is really the subject of another book – the reader is referred to *Pregnancy and Birth the Alexander Way* by Ilana Machover and Angela and Jonathan Drake (Robinson London, 1993) – but here is a brief résumé.

The Alexander Technique can provide – unlike any other approach – the means to achieve a better balance between the need to let instinctive forces drive labour and childbirth and yet to remain in conscious control. Especially from the second trimester onwards, body mechanics change rapidly. To help avoid low back pain produced by the growing bulge in front causing the back to sway (and the possibility of long-term back problems as habits formed in pregnancy often persist after the birth of the baby), it is important to begin Alexander lessons early in pregnancy, if not before. A secure understanding of how the body works can help short-circuit the pain-tension-more pain cycle which can interfere with the natural process of giving birth.

Gravity will assist in labour if the woman takes a more active role than is often encouraged, where the onus is on obstetric technology to deliver the baby. In the first stage of labour (dilation of the cervix) standing, walking about, lunging during contractions, kneeling and rocking on all fours (letting the head lead and the back to lengthen and widen), sitting in an expanded way over the sitting bones – all these ways of moving can help.

In the second stage (delivery), remembering to let the mouth soften as the woman breathes out, will help relax the pelvic floor. Facility in squatting, acquired in an unforced way during pregnancy or previously, provides an excellent position for giving birth; all fours is another possibility. Lying on the back is likely to interfere with birth (you wouldn't defecate with ease on your back!).

New parents are especially vulnerable to back problems. There are sleepless nights and many adjustments to make. Young children need carrying. An important thing to remember is that your legs provide you with the flexible base you need to adjust your position in response to the unpredictable load to lift and carry! To bend low enough to lift – especially if you cannot manage a low squat comfortably – use a half squat. Remember to let your lengthening spine and straightening legs make the lift, shoulders released as much as possible. You can then easily adjust your balance as needed (*Figs. 178–180*). Once you have lifted up the child, carry it close to your centre of gravity or in some kind of sling rather than carrying it on 'mother's hip', when the lower back will be badly twisted and swayed.

Gardening

Gardening is very demanding, especially for the office worker who gets carried away at the weekend. It is so easy to 'end-gain'. Whenever you think 'I must just finish that last border before I go in', is the time to stop and reconsider. *You may not feel the harm you are doing yourself at the time – pain is often delayed*.

There are many aids on the market now – long-handled tools, kneelers and so on – to

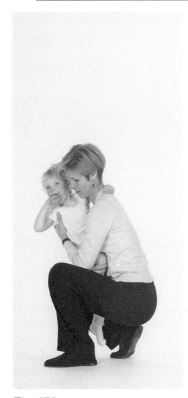

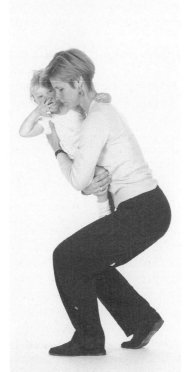

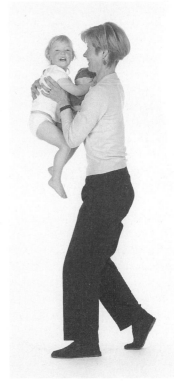

Fig. 178   *Fig. 179*   *Fig. 180*

mitigate some of the stresses of gardening. Don't stay in one position for very long. Pace yourself. Take frequent breaks; use the lie-down position more frequently – it will help you to acknowledge when you are beginning to overdo it!

The monkey and squat will be invaluable. A low lunge with the back heel sometimes lifted up off the ground is a useful flexible stance for digging. A tip when you need to turn out the spade or fork is to turn your whole body at the hips, adjusting your feet as necessary; if you merely turn the tool out to the side, you will almost certainly twist the back badly.

CHAPTER 10

Breathing and psychosomatics

The mechanics of breathing

Breathing is affected strongly by our emotions. Light, even breathing usually accompanies a calm state of mind. Sometimes we find ourselves holding our breath or breathing very fast and shallowly. This may happen when 'concentrating' on a difficult task or when we are nervous and afraid, and is associated with a general stiffening of the body.

Alexander's profound insight is that breathing occurs easily and naturally if we restore and maintain the proper length and width of the torso. The lowermost, 'floating' ribs are then free to move to allow the necessary lower chest expansion (about 70 per cent of lung capacity). On breathing in, the ribs move upwards and outwards. Not only is it a waste of effort to raise the upper chest when breathing at rest, but the hollowing and narrowing of the lower back actually reduces lung capacity. Breathing at rest is an activity which should take place at least as much by movement of the sides and back of the chest as of the front of the chest.

Alexander railed against the harmful effects of the deep breathing exercises which in his day were very much in vogue. Breathing exercises in various forms are still practised today in yoga, relaxation techniques, and some forms of therapy for example. Alexander's view was that we should not interfere directly with such a natural and spontaneous activity. What we should aim to do is to create the conditions which will allow breathing to take place freely and easily – by ensuring that the torso is properly lengthened and widened.

You might wish to experiment with what happens to your breathing when you deliberately disturb the NHB relationship. Raise your chest and hollow your lower back (*Fig. 181*). Put your hands round your waist at the back and at the sides. You will feel a little expansion at the sides of the chest, but virtually no movement at the back. To explore the other extreme, slump – rounding your back – and notice again that there is little movement of the lower back (*Fig. 182*). Somewhere in between these extremes, you should be able to feel more movement at the sides *and* back of the chest wall. The more the torso is allowed to lengthen and widen like an expanding cylinder, the more you will make the most of your lung capacity (*Figs. 183 and 184*).

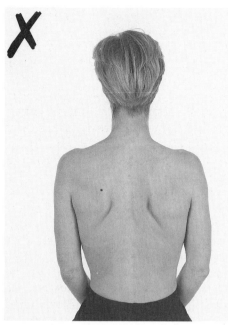

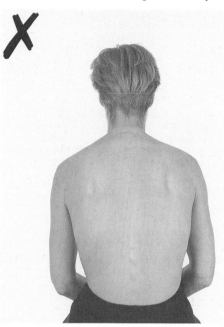

Fig. 181 Restricted breathing: raised chest and hollowed back.

Fig. 182 Restricted breathing: sunken chest and rounded back.

Figs. 183 and 184 A lengthened and widened torso allows breathing to take place by movement of the back and sides of the chest, as well as the front of the chest.

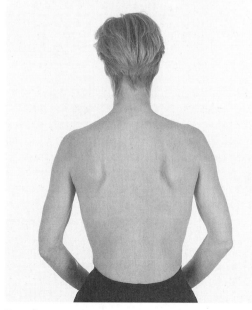

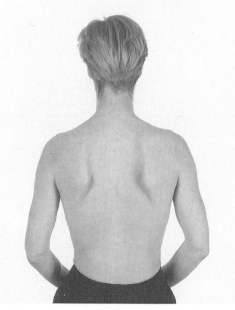

Breathing in.

Breathing out.

The whispered 'ah'

All the information Alexander had to go on at the beginning of his investigations was his tendency to suck in air between phrases. You can often hear this on radio and TV when microphones are placed close to the speaker; breathing in is accompanied by a gasping in of air – as in Alexander's case – and the head tends to jerk back, the chest to raise and the lower back to hollow (*Fig. 185*). Breathing out involves the opposite movements.

As Alexander's powers of observation developed, he noticed these contractions in his body not only when reciting but also, to a lesser degree, when speaking. In fact, if you watch anyone opening their mouth – in brushing the teeth, laughing, coughing, yawning and so on – it is as if the jaws have to be *prised* apart. If you make a big yawn, you will almost certainly observe your head pulling back and your chest raising.

Alexander therefore devised a procedure to *allow* his mouth to open in order to make a whispered sound without the usual tensions. This whispered 'ah' is a pre-requisite for any kind of vocalization. It is a very valuable procedure for any kind of public speaking and for people who tend to stutter or feel tense in social conversation. Again, this procedure needs to be introduced by your teacher (*Fig. 186*).

Any any stage of the procedure, if stiffening of the neck or downward pull of the head into the shoulders takes place – forwards or backwards – do not push on to the next stage, but stop and start again. It is an exercise not in 'end-gaining', but in attending to the 'means-whereby' the whispered sound may be made. Remember the need for inhibition, non-doing and direction-sending at each stage, and to maintain the length and width of the torso throughout this procedure. The full version of the whispered 'ah' is given first:

1) Let the tip of the tongue *loll* against the top of the lower teeth, a neutral, relaxed position for the tongue. (One of the first speech sounds a baby makes is 'ga ga'.) The teeth should be slightly apart from each other.

2) Smile a gentle smile, upper lip away from teeth; it helps if you can manage to think of something amusing (Alexander apparently used to say that if you couldn't, you might as well pack up and go home until you could!). The purpose of the smile is to help release tension in the facial muscles and to open the throat.

3) Let the lower jaw ease forward a little with the tongue gently directing it and then let it fall wide open as effortlessly as possible. Gravity will assist when in an upright position. (Take care not to pull the head down into the shoulders.)

Fig. 185 Sucking in air while speaking, tensing the throat and jerking back the head.

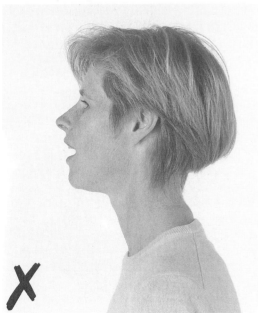

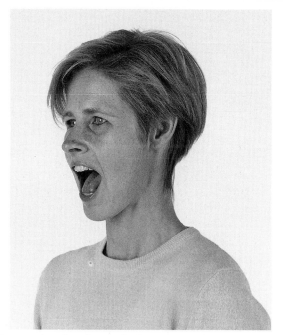

Fig. 186 The whispered 'ah'.

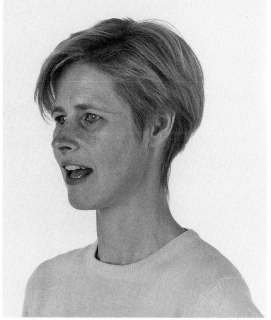

Fig. 187 The muted whispered 'ah'.

4) Whatever air you happen to have in your lungs, let it out with a whispered 'ah' sound. Listen to the sound you make. It should be smooth, full and even – not forced, thin or rasping.

5) Let the mouth close and let air come in through the nose.

6) Repeat a few times, aiming to do less and less muscular work each time. Be prepared to stop and start again if you get into any kind of difficulty.

A muted version of the whispered 'ah' can be done in public without any embarrassment! It is useful to practise a few of these before a public speaking engagement, whether to a large audience or a stressful meeting with someone. Let a faint smile play on your face, the tongue loll against the top of the lower teeth, let the mouth fall open a small distance and make an almost inaudible whispered 'ah' (*Fig. 187*).

You may find the whispered 'ah' easier at first while in the lying-down releasing position. Unnecessary movement of the head can be readily monitored on the books. The drawbacks are that you do not have gravity's assistance in opening the jaw and that the vocal cords are in a less advantageous position than when you are upright. You can practise the whispered 'ah' when standing or sitting. Monkey position is also an excellent way because the extra widening of the back facilitates breathing.

Some people have tremendous problems with jaw tension and even grind their teeth, especially at night. This is often associated with severe headaches and neck and shoulder problems and damage to teeth. The Technique should help enormously in those circumstances, but it is worth bearing in mind that if the teeth do not approximate accurately with the jaw closed, reflexes are triggered to cause teeth-grinding; and inhibition, when asleep, is impossible![1]

Practising the whispered 'ah' in monkey

This usually involves going into monkey and then putting the hands on the chair-rail (*Figs. 188–190*). The teacher will show you exactly how to go about this. Another possibility – from a standing position, feet a hips-to-shoulders-width apart – is to place the hands one by one onto the back of the chair; this can help you keep your back back as you lengthen along your spine to let your knees bend. You can then let your elbows move gently apart and away from your hips and lower back as you let your knees bend forward and away from each other. This procedure is basically an amalgam of two other procedures – monkey and hands on the chair-rail – which should be reviewed. You can then practise a few whispered 'ahs', giving particular attention to the lengthening and widening of the torso. This procedure, therefore, aims to encourage the proper relationship between neck, head and back, the appropriate separation of the limb joints away from each other and the release of the jaw.

Vocalization

From the whispered 'ah' you can go on to rehearse vowel sounds, as part of a tuning of the voice. It is also worth checking the pitch of your voice. Men often pitch the voice too low, women often pitch it too high; the consequences are strain and hoarseness with prolonged use. Many useful procedures to improve resonance and volume control – as well as other aspects of use of the voice – are suggested in Michael McCallion's *The Voice Book* (Faber and Faber, 1989).

Psychosomatics

The nature of the relationship between mind and body has been the subject of endless speculation in philosophy and theology, fuelled in recent years by advances in the

Fig. 188

Fig. 189

Fig. 190

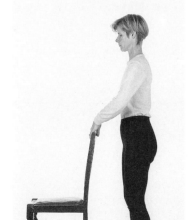
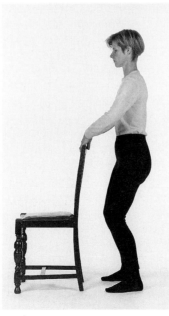
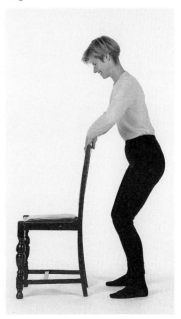

biological sciences and psychology, computer sciences and theoretical physics. What is the nature of the interaction of our emotions and thoughts and the physical body? And what is the perspective of the Alexander Technique?

I suspect that if Alexander were alive today he would look askance at much 'New Age' thinking about the 'whole human'. He applied his commonsense, powers of observation and the highest human faculty – reason – to solving his own psychophysical difficulties; and he developed a method by which we might sort out ours. The American philosopher, John Dewey, and other students of Alexander, have found that the benefits of the Technique have not only been physical ones, but also include an increased ability to clarify and modify their thinking.

The origins of the Technique define its scope. You will recall the story of Alexander's search for a practical remedy for his vocal problems. He began by trying to find out what he was *doing* which was causing his difficulties. He did not – as far as is known – concern himself with the question: 'why is it that I have such a passionate desire to perform on the stage yet manage to frustrate my best efforts?' He sought answers to 'what?' and 'how?' questions rather than 'why?' questions – although he ventured his own views about the general causes of misuse in his books. (Interestingly, although his restored vocal mechanism finally stood up to the rigours of performance, he never pursued a career as an actor but instead promulgated the discoveries he had made!) Alexander did not concern himself with plumbing the emotional reasons for his disability. He tried to change the one thing he guessed he might have some conscious control over – his 'doing'. And he came to the conclusion that the physical could not be separated from the mental. The one aspect of the mind that commanded his interest, however, was the will or *intention*, which seemed to be the

immediate trigger for the muscular responses interfering with his functioning.

The body has its reasons

The Alexander Technique does not deal directly with the emotional life. Some people would argue this is a serious limitation. The body has its reasons; misuse has an emotional component, a meaning, a personal significance of which the individual may not be aware. Change the physical aspect without dealing with the underlying psychological problem and it will surface later in another form or in a re-emergence of the original misuse pattern. People may therefore, benefit from counselling or some form of psychotherapy as well as the Alexander Technique.

Since the work of Freud, Groddeck and Reich, therapists have continued to explore the links between repressed emotion and physical tensions.[2] Some claim to have mapped out links between certain parts of the body, emotional difficulties and disorders in functioning in those parts of the body.[3] Common expressions show these links: e.g. 'shrugging the shoulders', 'butterflies in the stomach', 'gritting your teeth', 'get off my back'.

There is certainly a complex interaction at work; mood affects muscle and muscle affects mood. For example, a person who becomes depressed may continue to be depressed even when the circumstances which led to the depression have passed. To encourage – where possible – a more expanded posture in such a person, may help them recover. (It is also important to acknowledge that the relationship between pupil and teacher can be as important as re-education of body use – part of what is known in medicine as the 'placebo effect'.)

The question of motivation also needs to be examined: whether I want to heal myself. The phenomenon of 'secondary gain' is well-known in psychotherapy. It identifies the fact that at a particular stage in a person's life, there may be more advantage in creating and maintaining certain symptoms – even a life-threatening disease – than in overcoming them. A recent account of this psychosomatic theory, pushed to its limits, is given by Harrison:

If you ask the person with cancer why he needs cancer, he will tell you that he doesn't need it, want it or like it. And of course, to his knowledge, he's being truthful . . . (But) if the same person with cancer is offered the option of surviving by confronting his greatest fears, in many cases he will choose the cancer. His decision either way is entirely honorable.[4]

This view seems to ignore important factors such as genetic, environmental and social causes – as well as bad luck. But it does raise the issue of whether it is necessary or desirable or even possible to tackle the basic fears – or other painful emotion – directly. Perhaps emotional 'manure' is sometimes best left to rot down and feed the creative development of a person.

The Alexander Technique does not, of course, offer the individual the sense of purpose or meaning in life which philosophy or religion or psychotherapy may provide. The Technique does offer, though, a common-sense, 'here and now', approach to life's difficulties which can help considerably in 'the daily round'. Each day brings the opportunity to work on ourselves through challenges to be met and tasks that need doing – even trivial ones. We have some measure of choice about how we respond to these demands and our understanding of the importance of inhibition can be a turning-point in helping us navigate our direction in life.

Many forms of misuse are associated with neurotic patterns of behaviour where there seems to be a lack of order in the person's life. Religion has helped to provide a meaningful structure to daily life for many people. Now some people feel the need to create their own sense of order. One approach to dealing with the neurosis of much modern living – which may have resonance for those drawn to the Technique – is the method of re-education developed by a Japanese psychiatrist, Morito, and popularized in the west by Reynolds.[5] The three basic precepts of this approach can be summarized thus:

1) do what needs to be done (no more, no less: procrastination leads to emotional disturbance);

2) be clear about what you intend (actions follow intentions);

3) accept your emotions (you can do little to influence them *directly*, except in a self-destructive way – for example, through drug-abuse – but they can change in time through (1) and (2).)

Poise develops through being in reasonable command of yourself. By applying the principles of the Alexander Technique you may find it easier to deal with the increasingly rapid pace of modern life and to create your own responses to it. A calmer, slightly more detached frame of mind develops. While you still experience the range of emotions, you may find yourself less thrown by life's ups and downs and more able to use your energy efficiently. The next chapter is about using Alexander's principles to approach the learning of new skills with confidence.

CHAPTER 11

Mastering skills

Exercise is bunk. If you are healthy you don't need it. If you are sick, you shouldn't take it.

Henry Ford (attributed)

Most people love to do exercises; they save thought and inner struggle.

Patrick Macdonald

Trying is only emphasizing the thing we know already.

F.M. Alexander

When at first you don't succeed, never try again – at least, not in the same way. Trying almost always involves excessive tension.

Patrick Macdonald

Acquiring and mastering even the simplest skills calls for the most extraordinarily complex mind/brain/muscle coordination. Fortunately we do not have to attend to all the complexity at once, otherwise we would be like the centipede, who, wondering which leg to put forwards first, ends up tripping itself up! Much can be left to patterns already laid down in the brain.

There are times, though, despite our best efforts, when we seem to get stuck in a groove or struggle to no avail to get the hang of a new skill. The Alexander Technique gives you the confidence of a concrete procedure which you can apply to help undo unwanted habits, acquire new skills and improve on familiar ones. When we feel badly about our competence we can cope better by engaging in purposeful behaviour. This gives us more information about ourselves and the world. We are then more likely to succeed in achieving some of our goals and therefore earn the self-esteem and the personal satisfaction which comes from gaining more self-control and autonomy.

Ends and means

Alexander in his writing and teaching drew a great deal of attention to the harmful effects of 'end-gaining'. What is meant by this is the compulsion to strive for a particular end – no matter what cost to ourselves in undue tension, waste of effort and lack of consistency in performance.

The conclusion Alexander came to was that it is frequently the *idea* of the end we hold in mind which needs changing. We are deluded in believing that we can change how we do things without changing our mental 'templates'. We need, therefore, to be clear not only about the end we want to achieve, but also to work out appropriate and economical means for achieving that end.

The psychological barrier to change is our need to be right often when we are not! If we are willing to be wrong and therefore find out what is actually happening, we can become more aware of how we might be interfering with the performance of a particular skill. Only then do we have the possibility of improving it (and being less wrong!).

Conditions for developing skill

1) *Create a clear idea of what you want to do.* If you have only a vague idea of what it is you want to achieve, your actions will be correspondingly vague. This is trial and error without any clear guiding purposes. (Athletes and sportspeople often use visualization techniques to enhance performance: they imagine what a perfectly-executed movement would be like and let that image guide their coordination.[1])

2) *Think out appropriate means to achieve your end.* Break down the skill you wish to master into its component parts. Practise these parts separately, and then integrate them into more complex wholes. Most of us will need to work on one aspect at a time: we usually try to accomplish too much at once.

3) *Before acting, be clear what you intend.* Your primary intention should be to maintain the NHB relationship and your secondary aim to give the directions necessary for the particular action to be undertaken.

4) *Perform the movement.*

5) *Monitor performance.* Be on the alert for an undue rise in tension in the neck and other parts of the body (you will find this difficult if you have not had Alexander lessons), and disturbances in breathing –

indications you are over-reaching yourself. Get feedback by the use of mirrors, video or from your teacher.

Exercises and their limitations

Alexander, as has already been said, was very much opposed to exercising *per se* – the mechanical repetition of certain movements. His argument was that exercising tends to promote the conditions already present. Faulty kinaesthetic feedback – which is bound to be an important feature of the malcoordination you are trying to remedy through exercising, still operates. Most people are not aware that as soon as they start moving in any way whatsoever, they increase tension in the neck. This leads to unnecessary tension throughout the body, undue pressure on joints and breathing disturbance, as well as indirect effects on other aspects of functioning.

Recent physiological research has shown that voluntary muscle fibres can be divided into two types: red and white. Red fibres tend to be utilized in maintaining postural tone. They are also the fibres which tend to fire during slow, rhythmical activity. Distance runners tend to have a higher preponderance of red muscle fibres in their physique. These red fibres are linked to a slow centre in the brain governing movement. In contrast, white muscle fibres are linked to a fast centre in the brain; sprinters tend to have a greater proportion of white muscle fibres in their musculature. White muscle fibres are responsible for quick, powerful movement – but fatigue quickly.

It may seem logical to exercise and use the musculature not in play in the working day during your leisure time. However, for anyone with a sedentary lifestyle to work out in a gym or to do very vigorous forms of exercise – aerobics, squash and so forth – can be counter-productive. The emphasis will be on developing the white muscle fibres which will usurp the function of the red muscle fibres in postural support. The consequence will be to slump after a short while of sitting at a desk as the white muscle fibres fatigue.

Inexpensive forms of exercise more suitable for the office worker – which have the least potential for harm and some potential for good, intelligently carried out – include walking, cycling, swimming and T'ai Chi. You may also want to find out about an approach pioneered by Timothy Gallwey for improving performance at tennis called the 'inner game' (it has also been extended to golf, skiing and music), which has some interesting parallels with the Technique.[2]

Swimming

Swimming will be discussed in some detail – drawing on the conditions already outlined for developing skill based on Alexander principles. There is a cautionary note in relation to swimming: it is hardly the most natural form of exercise for us – we would have webbed feet and hands if that were the case! And done badly, it tends to over-develop the posterior musculature, which does not need any further emphasis. However, if you know how to swim efficiently on your front – and can balance that with swimming on your back – swimming is one of the most enjoyable and potentially beneficial forms of exercise. It might also aid personal survival; and it is suitable for any age and particularly for someone with joint problems.

I used to be one of those somewhat reluctant people seen in public swimming pools. My head would pull back out of the water (as if more concerned with keeping my hair dry!) and I made the wide sweeping arm movements of a laboured breaststroke. It occurred to me after I had completed my

training to be a teacher of the Alexander Technique that I would like to be able to enjoy the pleasures of swimming in an easy 'relaxed' way. And so I began to apply the principles of the Technique to improving my swimming. I can now swim front crawl and back crawl too, more or less to my satisfaction.

In the learning of any skill, it can be very difficult to apply the specific instructions of 'experts' to one's own experience. What follows, then, is an account of the key insights along the way which made all the difference to my own progress in swimming and which can be generalized to other skills.

First steps
Begin by creating a clear image of the stroke you wish to start learning (the 'end'). Watching others can help you begin to see what is required – and, most importantly, what is not required. This helped me considerably in learning front crawl; but it was not until I saw underwater film of a famous swimmer in action – slowed down – that I began to understand the actual movement of the arm reaching forward and the bent arm pull underneath the body. Above the surface of the water it is difficult to see what is going on underneath! Only exceptional swimming instructors are prepared to get into the water and demonstrate properly.

Having created a clear picture of your goal, the next step is to think out how you can work towards achieving it (the 'means-whereby'). The important realization for me was that, although I had had swimming lessons as a child – which had taught me to struggle through the water – I was still basically afraid of drowning! Over-stimulation of fear reflexes produces a form of 'startle response' where the neck stiffens and breathing and coordination is impaired. Through my increased ability to monitor undue tension in my body, it was quite

Fig. 191 The releasing glide: prerequisite for swimming on the front.

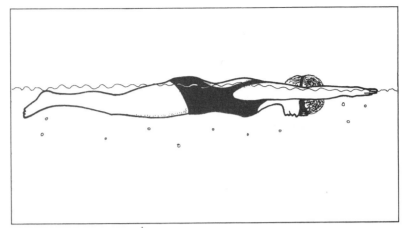

apparent that in many ways I was not allowing the water – and as water becomes saltier, buoyancy is increased – to support me.

The releasing glide

The primary control is of paramount importance in any movement; and the positioning of the head influences the alignment of the rest of the body in the water. If the head pulls back in front swimming strokes – apart from its effect of impairing coordination and breathing – the body position in the water is lowered and therefore resistance to movement through the water is increased.

In the swimming pool, gently kick off from the side with the arms straight out in front in order to glide a little way on the surface of the water. If you allow the head to be completely supported by the water, you will find that there is little tension in the neck and the eyes will more or less look straight down to the bottom of the pool (Fig. 191). This releasing position for the head, neck and torso – from which the specific arm and leg movements for breaststroke and front crawl are made – is the core 'non-doing' from which excessive increases in tension can be monitored as you practise the various aspects of the stroke.

Now the obvious problem to overcome is the face in the water and the need to breathe while swimming! The solution to this, unless your eyes are completely comfortable in the water, is to use a good pair of well-adjusted goggles. They will stop you screwing up your eyes (which lends itself to undue tension elsewhere). By wearing goggles you will be able to see where you are going, so that there is less reason to be afraid of the water.

Take a breath, kick off from the side of the pool, letting the head be supported by the water (you will be looking downwards) and blow bubbles. It is essential to be comfortable with this releasing glide before trying to go any further in learning to swim on the front. Then work on one aspect of the stroke at a time.

Breaststroke arm pull

The next stage in breaststroke is to master the breathing. The correct arm pull is crucial, because it is the arm pull which will produce the necessary clearance of the head out of the water to permit undisturbed breathing to take place. It should not be the old wide sweep to the side – a very inefficient stroke anyway.

Bear in mind that the correct sequence in breaststroke is *Kick – Glide – Pull*. Push off

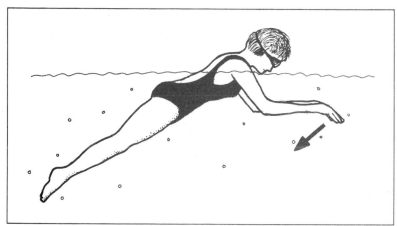

Fig. 192 Correct arm pull in breaststroke facilitates breathing.

from the side, the arms extended in front; and then turn the palms outwards and down, wrists flexing slightly, to pull you forwards and somewhat out of the water, as if you are lifting yourself up onto the top of a wall (*Fig. 192*). (The hands then come back together for the next glide, as if to 'clap your hands').

You will know that you are on the right lines when you observe the level of water – on the glide somewhere at the crown of your head – dropping to slightly below chin level as you pull yourself forwards and slightly out of the water. Notice that the head does not need to pull back *at all*. There will be a slight increase in tone in the neck muscles because less of the head is supported by the water during the arm pull. If you habitually hold the head out of the water, there will be an almost irresistible urge to pull the head even further back out of the water when you need to take a breath. This is where inhibition is so necessary. Repeat, reminding yourself not to be concerned at all – at this stage – with taking a breath while making the stroke.

Aim to do as little muscular work as possible. Practise two or three strokes at a time on one breath, breathing out steadily during the strokes; stop, breathe in, kick off and repeat the arm pull.

The next step is to let the jaw fall open as the water comes to just below chin level following the arm pull. Build up a consistent stroke so that no water gets into the mouth – *but without pulling back*! (Remember how frequently the pattern is to jerk back the head when taking a breath in normal circumstances!)

In that way, my old habit of pulling back my head to take a breath lessened. I was eventually able to take in air without any disturbance of the NHB relationship. If I reverted to my old habits, I didn't try to press on with another aspect of the stroke, but I would go back to the previous stage. After I had been following on my own this stop-start way of practising for some months, friends would remark – not quite knowing what I was doing – 'you must be super fit now: how many lengths can you swim?'!

The most efficient leg kick in breaststroke is to bend the legs to bring the feet to the buttocks and then turn the feet out sideways and kick backwards. If you bend the knees to the stomach, water resistance is increased by the thighs. At the same time, avoid arching the lower back as you bend the knees, even if you lose a little power in the kick.

Front crawl

In front crawl, avoid any tendency to pull the head back as you roll it to the side; this destabilizes the stroke and interferes with your coordination. Again, incorporate breathing in stages. Practise by allowing the head to roll to one side in the water as the arm on the other side begins to pull. Look out for objects at the side of the pool directly opposite your head position, so that you can readily see whether you are pulling the head backwards. Turn the head sufficiently in order for the mouth to clear the water. Then let it roll back to the neutral position, eyes looking down to the bottom of the pool. As before, consistently practise letting the mouth open without taking water in, *before attempting to take a breath*. Always be prepared to go back to the previous stage if you overextend yourself. Then master breathing on the other side as well so that you can breathe bilaterally on each third stroke.

Backstroke

It is a good idea to learn some form of backstroke so that you can balance the time swimming on your front with time on your back. This helps prevent over-development of the posterior musculature. People with shoulder injuries or as they get older often find the arm movements difficult in classic backstroke because of shoulder stiffness. There are other possibilities such as sculling with the arms or letting them enter the water wider than is usually recommended. With stiffness in shoulder joints, we may feel (faulty kinaesthetic awareness!) that the arms are entering the water straight – necessary to maximize the arm pull – when in fact they are bending, elbows touching the water first. It is preferable to have the arms entering the water at, say, two and ten o'clock, little fingers first so that an early 'catch' is made. You will probably need to turn your head momentarily on occasion when practising, to see whether what you feel you are doing is actually the case – or get an observer to tell you at which o'clock your arms are entering the water and whether they are in fact straight (but of course not rigid).

T'ai Chi Chu'an

If there is a form of exercise which can encourage good body use, then it is probably T'ai Chi. It was originally a martial art – the softest one. Its main use nowadays is as a form of ideal movement suitable for people of all ages.

There are fascinating parallels between T'ai Chi and the Alexander Technique. The means are different but a similar quality of coordination is aimed at. One of my Alexander pupils described T'ai Chi as a pure expression of the Alexander Technique in movement, and I believe she was right.

In T'ai Chi classic texts, descriptions of the requisite physical posture are as follows: 'holding the head as if suspended by a string from above, the entire body will feel light and nimble'; 'the depressing of the chest and the lifting of the back'; 'the loosening of the waist'. What is this if not pointing to the importance of the primary control? 'Direct the movement by using the will'. What is this if not Alexandrian direction? And the concept of *wu-wei* in Taoism appears similar to Alexandrian 'non-doing' (*Figs. 193 and 194*).

The language is poetic and uses images from nature. 'Your body should be so light and nimble that a feather could not land on it without being felt, and a fly could not alight on it without setting it in motion.' What T'ai Chi does not seem explicitly to identify is the unreliability of kinaesthetic perception and its harmful consequences for repetition of movement. It also lacks the rigour of the concept of inhibition and a precise understanding of the primary control which the Alexander Technique – properly learnt – supplies. In T'ai Chi classes you can see poor coordination repeated again and again. T'ai Chi could be learnt more efficiently by applying Alexander principles to the form. At the same time, the form – the sequence of movements in T'ai Chi – is an opportunity to test and develop your understanding of the principles of well-coordinated movement. For the student of the Alexander Technique, T'ai Chi provides a laboratory and a training ground for the kinds of ways the body should be used in everyday life. In particular, for those of us who for years have made top-heavy bending movements, the practice of T'ai Chi – properly undertaken – can help restore the supple and powerful use of the legs we had as young children.

The preparation and performance of music

The Alexander Technique helps sort out the bad backs and the repetitive strain injuries from which musicians frequently suffer; and it is also an important discipline in the preparation and performance of music.

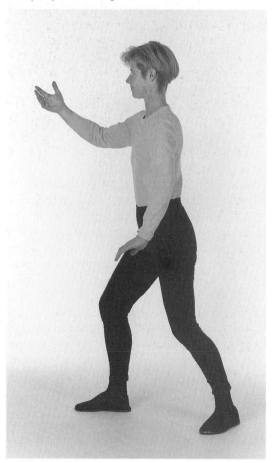

Fig. 193 T'ai chi, showing use of the 'lunge'.

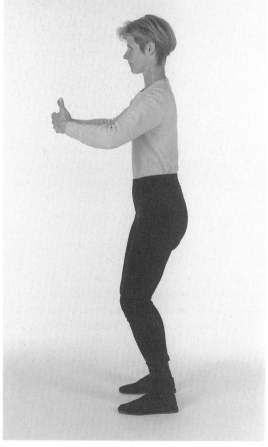

Fig. 194 Chi kung: use of the monkey.

Fig. 195 Artur Rubinstein, 1887–1982. Perfectly poised in performance. (Photo: Rex Features)

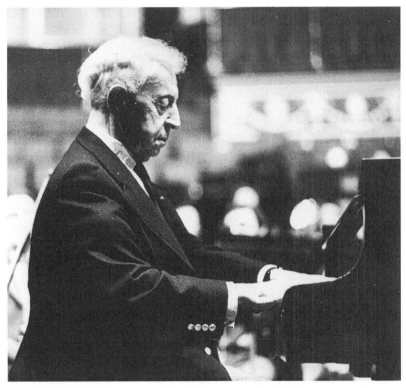

Nelly Ben-Or, professor of piano at the Guildhall School of Music and Drama in London, and Alexander teacher, describes the clarity of approach that the Technique can give musicians.[3] She emphasizes the need to thoroughly understand the music (as a conductor studies the score) before going anywhere near the instrument. If the music is clear in your mind, then your muscles have the best possible chance of responding properly. She explains how a passage labelled 'difficult' – perhaps because it needs to be played very fast or very loudly – becomes difficult because of the mental block created and because the musician tries to substitute muscular overwork (and misuse) for the intelligent preparation of the music in his or her mind.

Practice does not guarantee perfection. On the contrary, we can rehearse the very things we should be avoiding. The pianist Rubinstein was said to practise for no longer than two hours – worth seven or eight hours of anyone else's practice. He also used to do entirely the wrong thing just before going onto the concert platform; for instance playing a scale in C major on one hand and C minor in the other; his justification was that he couldn't possibly play as bad as that when he was on stage! As Alexander observed: 'To know when we are wrong is all we shall ever know in this world.'

Afterword

The aim of *The Alexander Technique in Everyday Life* has been to help you understand the nature and causes of patterns of misuse which can adversely affect your functioning. It is important to appreciate the kind of change that is required. Many approaches which promise to improve your health often lead to a 'different kind of badly'. The 'body know-how' the Alexander Technique proposes is a more holistic approach that links aspects of the mind and body in a precise way. The more you understand about the Technique, the more you realize you are not dealing with 'physical culture', so much as a process of clarifying your intentions. Your general coordination can then improve.

Alexander said that if anyone did exactly what he did, then they would not need a teacher. Most of us are not prepared to take on the enormous mental work that Alexander did. Fortunately we did not need to do so – to anything like the same extent. He – and the teachers he trained – can teach you in a relatively small number of lessons what it took him years to work out for himself.

Where can I go from here?

There are some things you can begin doing straight away, such as daily lying down and thinking about the various ergonomic improvements you can make. You might like to read further about the Technique, and suggestions are given on page 139. The author's *Introductory Guide to the Alexander Technique* is a useful overview. The first chapter of Alexander's *Use of the Self*, 'Evolution of the Technique' is highly recommended.

At the same time, we need to understand that even following the guidance of a teacher, the urge to 'end-gain' on our own can still be very powerful. We so much want to get it right all at once; or other aspects of our lives assume higher priority and the importance of primary control is easily forgotten in the rush of daily living!

We will need a teacher – and sometimes a different teacher at another stage – to get us properly started and help us on the way. The real work, though – finally – is what we make our own. Macdonald recalled his boxing teacher saying to him as a boy in the ring one day, 'I can teach you to do this, but I can't learn you. You will have to learn yourself!'

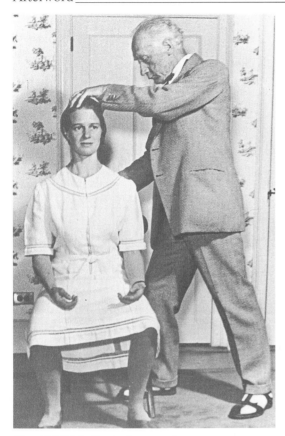

Fig. 196 F.M. Alexander at work

introductory lesson or two from two or three teachers – if that option is open to you – and then decide with whom to continue.

Frequency of lessons

Alexander often used to see people daily over a few weeks for a basic course of lessons. He had, by all accounts, great skill in the use of his hands and could produce remarkable change in people – even those with severe disabilities – in a relatively short time. In my opinion an ideal frequency of lessons is twice a week, initially. Some people can manage on one lesson a week; others need three a week for a while to make enough impact on chronic patterns. Your teacher will advise you on whether you would benefit from more frequent lessons. Sometimes it may be better to wait until you can really commit yourself to coming often enough to make it genuinely worthwhile.

You will probably need lessons over two or three months to establish a sound basis for continual self-development, although some people learn enough to get some relief from their particular problem in a matter of weeks.

Choosing a teacher

More and more teachers are being trained to teach the Alexander Technique. The Society of Teachers of the Alexander Technique and equivalent bodies in other countries – from whom lists of teachers can be obtained (see Appendix 2) – regulate the three year training courses for teachers. As with all other professions, the quality of individual teachers varies. It is also partly a matter of personality whether you respond to a certain teacher – and that may alter as your understanding grows.

My advice to someone seeking a teacher is to go mainly by personal recommendation. It can sometimes be helpful to take an

What happens in a lesson

In a lesson a competent teacher will convey, through the use of his or her hands, the improved body use that is required. This should be directly linked with the 'thinking in activity' – inhibition and non-doing and direction-sending – which should be your conscious participation in the lesson. This thinking in activity should increasingly replace the teachers' hands when you are on your own.

The lesson (which normally lasts 30–45 minutes) will probably include chair work, other procedures, some table-work – the releasing lying down position described earlier – and the rest might be spent in application.

Notes

Introduction

1) Details of Dr Wilfred Barlow's research can be found in accessible form in his book *The Alexander Principle* and *More Talk of Alexander* (edited).

2) Alexander does give some practical guidance on: standing, walking and getting in and out of a chair in *Man's Supreme Inheritance*, part II, VII; ploughing(!) *ibid*, pp. 143–5; golf, *ibid*, pp. 127–8, pp. 133–6 and in *The Use of the Self*, Ch 3, 'The Golfer Who Cannot Keep His Eyes on the Ball'.

1. What is good body use?

1) Feldenkrais M. *Awareness Through Movement*, Penguin, 1980. Feldenkrais derived many of his ideas from Alexander.

2. The primary control

1) Tinbergen N., 'Ethology and Stress Disease' (Nobel Prize Oration), *Science*, 185, 1974; pp. 22–7, also reprinted in Barlow's *More Talk of Alexander*.

During a lecture that David Garlick gave at the International Congress of Alexander Teachers in Brighton, 1988, he mentioned how he came to be interested in researching the Technique – through reading Tinbergen's Nobel Prize Oration. When Garlick went to meet Tinbergen at Oxford University – some years later – he discovered that he was the *first scientist* to express an interest in Tinbergen's remarks! (Much could be written about the fact that Alexander cannot be pigeon-holed into any kind of academic framework; and that much scientific enquiry is made in fairly predictable directions.)

2) Garlick D. (ed), *Proprioception, Posture and Emotion*, Committee in Postgraduate Medical Education, University of New South Wales, 1982.

3. How to change

1) Alexander F.M., *Man's Supreme Inheritance*, p. 31.

2) Libet B., 'Unconscious cerebral initiative and the role of the conscious will in voluntary activity', *The Behavioural and Brain Sciences*, 8, 1985, p. 9.

3) Macdonald P.J., 'On Giving Directions, Doing and Non-Doing', 1963. Alexander

Memorial Lecture printed in *The Alexander Journal*, 9, 1988, pp. 4–11. Also published in his book, *The Alexander Technique: As I See It*, Rahula Books, 1989.

4) *Ibid*, p. 64.

4. Applying Alexander principles to everyday activities

1) Conable, B. & W., *How to Learn the Alexander Technique*, Andover Road Press, Columbus, Ohio, 1992 (can be ordered through STAT books – see *Further Reading*).

5. On the importance of lying down

1) D'Arcy Thompson, from 'On Growth and Form', quoted in F.P. Jones, *Body Awareness in Action*.

6. Keeping your head

1) Jones F.P., *Body Awareness in Action*, pp. 158–9. Schocken Books, 1988.

2) Barnes J., *Improve Your Eyesight: A Guide to the Bates Method*, Angus & Robertson, 1987: a good up-to-date guide.

7. Legging it

1) Tinbergen N., *Use and Misuse in Evolutionary Perspective*, 1976 Alexander Memorial Lecture, printed in Barlow W. (ed)., *More Talk of Alexander*.

2) *Orthotics* concerns itself with body mechanics and the disturbances created by imbalances in the feet and lower limbs. To correct these through appropriate support to the feet can, in certain cases, make it easier to restore the proper working of the primary control. A practitioner specializing in orthotics can be found through your local chiropodist.

8. Your ischial tuberosities

1) Alexander F.M., *Constructive Conscious Control of the Individual*, Part II, Chapter IV, Illustration.

10. Breathing and psychosomantics

1) People who habitually grind their teeth often have neck and shoulder problems and headaches, as well as dental and gum problems. It is worth considering an expensive dental procedure – 'equilibration' – which involves shaving microns off appropriate teeth so that all the teeth approximate adequately when the jaw is closed. In selected cases, it can produce much improvement and soon pays for itself by avoiding costly crowns!

2) See, for instance, Groddeck's *The Book of the It*, Vision Press, 1979. He used massage and would direct his attention to the emotional aspects of particular physical symptoms or, if the complaint was of psychological disturbance, he was at least as interested in the physical manifestations of the person's illness. Note also the concept of 'character-armouring' of Wilhelm Reich and the bio-energetic school, for example Alexander Lowen, Stanley Keleman.

3) See, for instance: Hay L., *Heal Your Body*, Hay House, 1982; Harrison J., *Love Your Disease: It's Keeping You Healthy*, Angus & Robertson, 1984.

4) *Ibid*, p. 277.

5) Reynolds D.K., *Playing Ball on Running Water*, Sheldon, 1985.

11. Mastering skills

1) Syer C., Connolly C., *Sporting Body, Sporting Mind*, Cambridge University Press, 1984.

2) Gallwey W.T., *The Inner Game of Tennis*, Pan, 1974. See also Green B., with Gallwey, *The Inner Game of Music*; Gallwey W.T., *The Inner Game of Golf*, *The Inner Game of Skiing* – all in Pan paperback.

3) Ben-Or Nelly, *The Alexander Technique in the Preparation and Performance of Music*, Alexander Memorial Lecture 1987; booklet available from STAT Books.

Ergonomic suggestions

It cannot be said often enough that the workstation should be arranged to allow optimal functioning: we do not need any encouragement to distort ourselves to the demands of work!

A working chair should not only be adjustable in respect of height, but also in respect of tilt of the seat pad. Ideally we should learn to support our own backs entirely; for most of us, however, a back pad, adjustable against the lower/middle back – even in a slightly forward tilting position – is highly desirable. In addition, if the whole chair can rock gently to and fro, some of the deleterious effects of static posture can be mitigated. The following table is intended as a *very rough* guide to chair/desk relativity for particular tasks:

Person	Chair (sitting bones to floor)	Desk/ writing	Desk/ keyboard
60/152	18/46	>28/71	<24/61
64/163	20/51	>30/76	<26/66
68/173	22/56	>32/81	<28/71
72/183	24/61	>34/86	<30/76
76/193	26/66	>36/91	<32/81

Recommended chair/desk heights (approximate in inches/centimetres)

A working chair should tilt by about 4–5 degrees. If you are trying to modify an ordinary dining chair, most people will need their sitting cushion not only to tilt them slightly forward but also to raise them up a little. If you want to make your own, here are some suggestions. You will need dense chip-foam – CM6–9lb topped with ½"/1cm TP40 for comfort, cut 15"/38cm wide by 14"/35cm long to fit an ordinary dining chair. To raise an 18"/48cm chair for your height and to provide a 4–5 degree angle, the following approximate measurements for the wedge shape apply:

5'2"–5'6"/157–168cm, 2.25"/6cm–>0.75"/2cm;

5'6"–5'10"/168–178cm, 3"/7.5cm–>1"/2.5cm;

5'10"–6'2"/178–183cm, 4"/10cm–>1/4"/3.5cm.

The foam will need to be covered. (Some of the organizations listed in Appendix 3 have these cushions for sale.)

Design of writing slope

The writing surface (approximately 20 inches/50cm wide by 17 inches 42.5cm long) should slope by about 15–18 degrees. Such a slope can be constructed using birch-wood ply (which will give a hard, smooth surface). Fix a very small ledge on the bottom edge to stop paper or books sliding off. If it is angled with another piece of ply attached by means of a strip of piano hinge, the slope can readily be folded away and stored flat when not in use. Small rubber feet under this edge and the front edge will prevent the slope from sliding on the surface of the desk. It can be finished off with a matt varnish. Again, some of the organizations listed will sell similar designs.

Alexander Technique professional societies

The following societies will provide a list of teachers of the Alexander Technique who have completed the three years of an approved training course (please send a stamped addressed enveloped):

United Kingdom

The Society of Teachers of the Alexander Technique (STAT)
20 London House
266 Fulham Road
London SW10 9EL
Tel: 0171 351 0828
(They also have a catalogue of books for sale on the Technique.)

Australia

Australian Society of Teachers of the Alexander Technique (AUSTAT)
PO Box 716
Darlinghurst
NSW 2025
Tel: 008 339 571

Canada

Canadian Society of Teachers of the Alexander Technique (CANSTAT)
Box 47025
Apt. 12–555
West 12th Avenue
Vancouver BC V5Z 3XO
Canada

Denmark

Danish Society of Teachers of the Alexander Technique (DFLAT)
Mark Crue
OHO Ruds Gade 38st. th.,
DK-8200
Aarhus N
Denmark

Germany

German Society of the Teachers of the Alexander Technique (GLAT)
Postfach 5312
79020 Frieburg
Germany
Tel: 0761 383357

Israel

Israeli Society of Teachers of the Alexander Technique (ISTAT)
c/o Gideon Avrahami
Kibbutz Ein-Shemer
M.P. Menashe 37845
Israel
Tel: 06 374196

The Netherlands

Netherlands Society of Teachers of the Alexander Technique
Postbus 15591
1001 NB Amsterdam
The Netherlands
Tel: 020 625 3163

South Africa

35 Thornhill Road
Rondebosch 7700
South Africa
Tel: 021 686 8454

Switzerland

Swiss Society of Teachers of the Alexander Technique (SVLAT)
Postfach
CH-8032
Zurich
Switzerland

United States

North American Society of Teachers of the Alexander Technique (NASTAT)
PO Box 517
Urbana
IL 61801–0517
USA

There are also qualified teachers in many other countries. You can find out about teachers not represented by a national body through the UK Society of Teachers of the Alexander Technique.

Organizations selling chairs and posture aids

ADVANCE SEATING designs

Unit 7
Everitt Rd
London NW10 6PL
Tel: 0181 961 4515
Alan and Lesley Glaser assess each client and advise on the appropriate chair from their excellent 'Opera' range; seats and backs are designed for specific postural problems. They can also supply industrial seating and bespoke office seating for a wide range of disabilities.

Alternative Sitting

PO Box 101
Witney
Oxfordshire
OX8 7WZ
Tel: 01993 700280
David Robinson takes a great deal of trouble to work out the best solution for clients who wish to improve their sitting at work.

BACK-IN-ACTION™

PO Box 1457
Bourne End
Bucks SL8 5YU
Tel: 01628 527659
A company which provides postural advice, as well as selling a wide range of products, with showrooms in Marlow and central London.

Positive posture

120 Church Lane
London N2 0TB
Tel: 0181 883 7828
Gill Jordan, physiotherapist, sells wedges, back rests, neck pillows and writing slopes at reasonable prices.

Pelvic Posture Ltd

Glaston Hill House
Glaston Hill Road
Eversley
Hampshire RG27 0LX
Tel: 01734 328087
John Gorman sells the simple working chair shown in some of the illustrations used in

this book, as well as chair pelvic support cushions and sitting wedges.

Posture point

Logierait
Links Way
Thurlton
Norwich
Norfolk NR14 6RF
Tel: 01508 548 928
Fiona Marlow sells a wide range of chairs and accessories.

J. Drake

247 College Rd
Norwich
Norfolk NR2 3JD
Tel: 01603 503794

I have chair and car wedges and writing slopes available at reasonable cost. (No postal service, unlike the other organizations listed.)

Uphold

Tel: 01225 743592
Book support allows reading while lying down.

Further reading

What follows is a selected list of books on the Alexander Technique. Many are available from STAT Books, 20 London House, 266 Fulham Rd, London SW10 9EL; some are out-of-print* but still worth reading if you can get hold of them through a library or second hand book-finding service.

Alexander F.M., Maisel E. (ed)., *The Essential Writings of F. Matthias Alexander*, Thames and Hudson, new ed. 1989. A compilation of Alexander's four books – including his account of the evolution of the Technique, the introductions to Alexander's books by John Dewey, some of Alexander's teaching aphorisms and a long introduction by the editor on Alexander and a history of the development of the Technique.

*Alexander F.M., *Man's Supreme Inheritance*, (1910). Centreline Press USA. The style of writing in all his books is verbose and repetitious. Good bedtime reading for insomniacs but there are gems to be found for committed students of Alexander!

Alexander F.M., *Constructive Conscious Control of the Individual*, (1923) Gollancz, 1986.

Alexander F.M., *The Use of the Self*, (1932) Gollancz, 1985. Chapter 1 is Alexander's account of the evolution of the Technique.

*Alexander F.M., *The Universal Constant in Living*, (1941) Centreline Press.

Barlow W., *The Alexander Principle*, Arrow, 2nd edn 1990. A good introductory book on the Technique by a former consultant in physical medicine who trained with Alexander.

*Barlow W. (ed), *More Talk of Alexander: Aspects of the Alexander Principle*, Gollancz, 1978. A treasury of short articles and reprinted lectures including Marjory Barlow's (Alexander's niece and distinguished teacher of the Technique) excellent account of the Technique.

Ben-Or N, *The Alexander Technique in the Preparation and Performance of Music* and *A Pianist's Thoughts on the Alexander Technique*. Booklet includes the 1987 Memorial Alexander Lecture; fascinating insights for all musicians, available from STAT Books.

Conable B.&W., *How to Learn the Alexander*

Technique, Andover Road Press, Columbus, Ohio, 1992.

Drake, J., *Introductory Guide to the Alexander Technique*, Thorsons, 1993.

*Fenton, J.V., *Choice of Habit*, MacDonald and Evans, 1973. Practical applications of the Technique in school

Garlick D., *The Lost Sixth Sense: A Medical Scientist Looks at the Alexander Technique*, University of New South Wales, 1990.

Gelb M., *Body Learning: An Introduction to the Alexander Technique*, Aurum Press, 3rd ed, 1994. A good synthesis of the basic concepts.

Gorman, D., *The Body Moveable*, 1981. Detailed account of the human musculoskeletal system, with reference to the Alexander Technique.

Gray, J., *Your Guide to the Alexander Technique*, Gollancz, 1990. A very useful account of how to work on yourself by a teacher trained by the Barlows.

*Jones F.P., *Body Awareness in Action*, Schocken Books, NY, 2nd ed 1988. A well-written account of the lives and work of F.M. Alexander and his brother by a classics scholar who became an Alexander Teacher, and who turned to experimental science to try to 'prove' the Technique.

Macdonald P.J., *The Alexander Technique: As I See It*, Rahula Books, 1989. Reflections by a master teacher.

Machover I., Drake A. & J., *Pregnancy and Birth the Alexander Way*, Robinson, 1993.

*Westfeldt L., *F. Matthias Alexander: The Man and His Work*, new ed Centreline Press. An inspiring story of how she helped herself overcome – to a large extent – the effects of childhood polio, aided by the Technique; and her observations on Alexander.

Index

Also available . . .

YOGA
Step by Step
CHERYL ISAACSON

Here is a fresh, clear look at the benefits that yoga has to offer *everyone*. By practising simple methods of moving, stretching and breathing, young bodies can stay supple and full of vitality, while older ones can shed aches and pains and even delay signs of ageing. Yoga can be a 'preventive medicine' as well as providing relief from existing problems. Young or old, male or female, healthy or infirm – there is something for everyone in the broad spectrum of rewards that yoga offers.

Cheryl Isaacson explains what yoga can do for *you* and how it works. She provides all the information you need to begin practising yoga, and gives details of warm-up exercises as well as guidance on yoga breathing. The 25 yoga postures described are fully illustrated, stage-by-stage, so that they can be performed correctly right from the start. And, special guidelines are given for children, the elderly and those with particular aims, to help maximise the benefits that yoga can bring.

MEDAU:
THE ART OF ENERGY
LUCY JACKSON
featuring
LALA MANNERS

'Medau is Magic' *Health and Fitness Magazine*
'Medau . . . the secret of a youthful body' *Harpers and Queen*
'Medau stretches the body in the most natural way' *Vogue*
'Medau . . . my favourite form of exercise' Diana Moran (The Green Goddess)
'Medau leaves you full of joy and vitality' Geraldine James (star of Jewel in the Crown)

What is Medau?

An exciting form of exercise which combines the rhythm of dance with natural whole body movement. It mixes aerobics and stretch – without straining the body. Whether you are 10, 20 or over 40 the movements can be done at the pace which is *right for you*.

The Art of Energy is a unique programme of Medau movements combining

• **Stretch** • **Strength** • **Stamina** • **Suppleness**

It will leave you fitter, leaner, healthier and full of confidence; and above all – it is enjoyable to do.

Medau Movement can be adapted for every need. Lucy Jackson shows you how to create a strong and healthy body for life.

So – *come alive* with Medau! Throw away your gruelling repetitive routines and learn to be in tune with your body – the natural way.

Medau is for everyone – Medau is for YOU.

LUCY JACKSON and LALA MANNERS are the dynamic mother and daughter team who teach Medau throughout the world. Their ART OF ENERGY workout is featured on MEDAU: THE ART OF ENERGY video available from Polygram.